Illustrated Clinical Cases:
ENT Medicine and Surgery

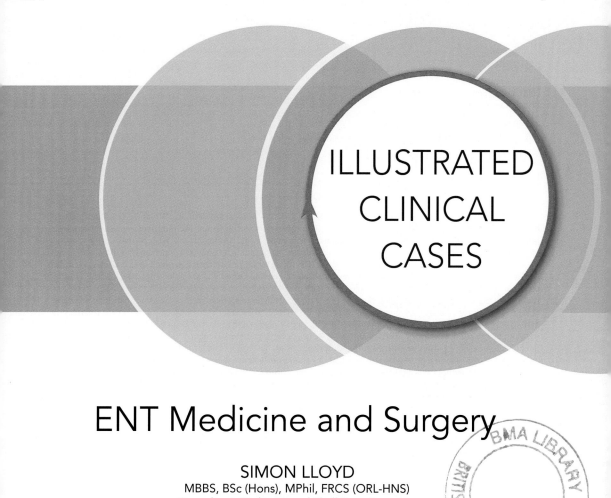

ILLUSTRATED CLINICAL CASES

ENT Medicine and Surgery

SIMON LLOYD
MBBS, BSc (Hons), MPhil, FRCS (ORL-HNS)
Consultant Otologist and Skull Base Surgeon
Manchester University NHS Foundation Trust;
Professor of Otolaryngology, University of Manchester, UK

MANOHAR BANCE
MBChB, MSc, FRCSC
Professor of Otology and Skull Base Surgery
University of Cambridge, UK

JAYESH DOSHI
MBChB (Hons), MMed, PhD, FRCS (ORL-HNS)
Consultant ENT Surgeon, Heartlands Hospital,
University Hospitals Birmingham NHS Foundation Trust;
Honorary Senior Clinical Lecturer, University of Birmingham, UK

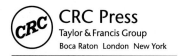

CRC Press
Taylor & Francis Group
Boca Raton London New York

CRC Press is an imprint of the
Taylor & Francis Group, an **informa** business

CRC Press
Taylor & Francis Group
6000 Broken Sound Parkway NW, Suite 300
Boca Raton, FL 33487-2742

Library of Congress Cataloging-in-Publication Data

Names: Lloyd, Simon (Simon Kinglsey Wickham), author. | Bance, Manohar, author. | Doshi, Jayesh, author.
Title: ENT medicine and surgery : illustrated clinical cases / Simon Lloyd, Manohar Bance, Jayesh Doshi.
Other titles: Illustrated clinical cases.
Description: Boca Raton : CRC Press, [2016] | Series: Illustrated clinical cases
Identifiers: LCCN 2016041239| ISBN 9781482230413 (pbk. : alk. paper) | ISBN 9781482230420 (eBook PDF)
Subjects: | MESH: Otorhinolaryngologic Diseases | Otorhinolaryngologic Surgical Procedures | Case Reports | Examination Questions
Classification: LCC RF56 | NLM WV 18.2 | DDC 617.5/1–dc23
LC record available at https://lccn.loc.gov/2016041239

**Visit the Taylor & Francis Web site at
http://www.taylorandfrancis.com**

**and the CRC Press Web site at
http://www.crcpress.com**

CONTENTS

Section 3: Otology and skull base

Section 4: Rhinology and facial plastics

Section 5: Paediatrics

Section 6: Miscellaneous

PREFACE

The ability to make an accurate diagnosis is the most important skill a clinician can possess. The key attributes in developing this skill are experience, knowledge and confidence. These are only acquired over time but the process can be facilitated through shared experiences.

This book is made up of a series of case studies covering all aspects otolaryngology from basic issues in otolaryngology to more challenging clinical cases. The aim of the book is to build a clinically relevant knowledge base for the reader through discussion of the clinical principles that each case elucidates.

It is aimed at practicing otolaryngologists, trainees and general practitioners who wish to develop their diagnostic skills in otolaryngology for the benefit of their patients. It also provides a useful aid for those undertaking post-graduate exams and facilitates continuing professional development.

We hope that this book will highlight important points in otolaryngology and provide an enjoyable means for clinicians to enhance their diagnostic skills in otolaryngology.

AUTHORS

Simon Lloyd, MBBS, BSc (Hons), MPhil, FRCS (ORL-HNS), is a professor of otology and skull base surgery at University of Manchester and consultant otolaryngologist at Manchester NHS Foundation Trust and Salford Royal NHS Foundation Trust in Manchester, United Kingdom.

Manohar Bance, MBChB, MSc, FRCSC, is a professor of otology and skull base surgery at University of Cambridge, United Kingdom.

Jayesh Doshi, MBChB (Hons), MMed, PhD, FRCS (ORL-HNS), is a consultant ENT surgeon at the Heart of England Foundation Trust, Birmingham, United Kingdom, and honorary senior clinical lecturer at University of Birmingham, United Kingdom.

CONTRIBUTORS

The authors wish to thank the following for their invaluable contributions to the case studies in this book:

Osama Al Hamarneh, MBBS, MD, FRCS (ORL-HNS)
Jordan Teaching Hospital and Medical Center
Amman, Jordan

Thomas Beech, MBChB, MSc, FRCS (ORL-HNS)
University Hospital Birmingham
Birmingham, United Kingdom

Rebecca Field, MBChB, FRACS (ORL-HNS)
Christchurch Hospital
Christchurch, New Zealand

Edward Flook, FRCS Ed (ORL-NHS)
Glan Clwyd Hospital
North Wales, United Kingdom

Amanda McSorley, MBChB (Hons), BSc (Hons), MRCS, DOHNS
North West Deanery
Manchester, United Kingdom

Abhijit Ricky Pal, MB, BChir, MA (Cantab), MD, FRCS (ORL-HNS)
Oxford University Hospitals NHS
    Foundation Trust
Oxford, United Kingdom

Glen J. Watson, FRCS (ORL-HNS), DOHNS, MBBCh
Royal Hallamshire Hospital
Sheffield, United Kingdom

Susannah Penney, MBChB, DOHNS, FRCS (ORL-HNS)
Manchester Royal Infirmary
Manchester, United Kingdom

Kay Seymour, MA (Cantab), MB, BChir, FRCS (ORL-HNS)
Barts Health, Royal London Hospital
London, United Kingdom

We would also like to thank the following people who helped to illustrate the cases:

Shahzada Ahmed, BSc (Hons), DLO, FRCS (ORL-HNS), PhD
University Hospitals Birmingham NHS Trust
Birmingham, United Kingdom

Shahram Anari, MD, MSc, FRCS (ORL-HNS)
Birmingham Heartlands Hospital
Birmingham, United Kingdom

Steve Colley, MBChB, FRCR
Queen Elizabeth Hospital Birmingham
Birmingham, United Kingdom

Ann Louise McDermott, FDSRCS, FRCS (ORL-HNS), PhD
Birmingham Children's Hospital
Birmingham, United Kingdom

Nicola Pargeter, BSc, MSc, RCSLT, Reg HCPC
Birmingham Heartlands Hospital
Birmingham, United Kingdom

Christopher Thomson, FRACS
Christchurch Hospital
Christchurch, New Zealand

Tim J. Woolford, MD, FRCS (ORL-HNS)
Manchester Royal Infirmary
Manchester, United Kingdom

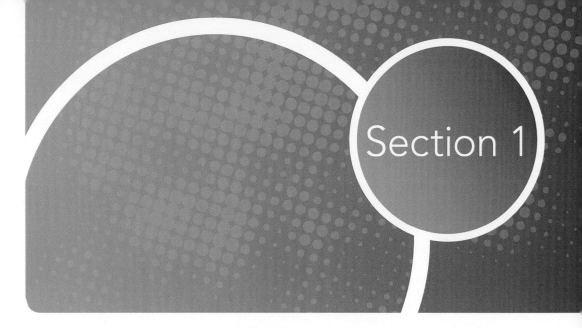

HEAD AND NECK

CASE 1

QUESTIONS 1

A 39-year-old male presents with a 2-month history of right throat pain. There is no significant past medical history and he is a lifelong non-smoker who drinks 20 units of alcohol per week. Examination of the neck reveals a 1 cm right level II lymph node. Examination of the oropharynx reveals the following:

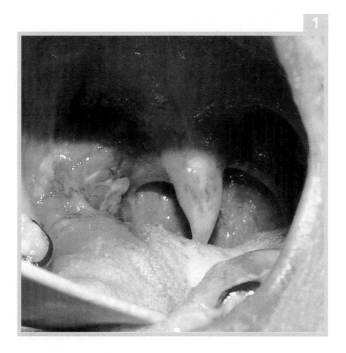

i.   What is the likely diagnosis?

ii.   What are the major risk factors for this condition?

iii.   How would you investigate this patient?

iv.   Outline the T staging classification for this condition.

v.   This patient has a TNM stage of T1, N1, M0. Outline the treatment options.

vi.   Should the N0 neck be treated in T1–T2 disease?

i.   The right tonsil is enlarged and ulcerated – it is likely to be a squamous cell carcinoma.

ii.   Smoking, alcohol, human papilloma virus (HPV) and betel nut chewing.

iii. Fine needle aspiration cytology (FNAC) of the neck node.

Magnetic resonance imaging (MRI) of neck – to assess primary tumour and cervical metastasis.

Computed tomography (CT) of thorax – for staging purposes.

Panendoscopy and biopsy for definitive histological diagnosis, HPV testing of biopsy specimen.

Tonsillectomy should not be carried out in the presence of obvious malignancy as this will limit the treatment option of future transoral laser surgery.

iv.   Tx: primary tumour cannot be assessed.

T0: no evidence of primary tumour.

Tis: carcinoma *in situ*.

T1: tumour 2 cm or smaller in the greatest dimension.

T2: tumour larger than 2 cm but 4 cm or smaller in the greatest dimension.

T3: tumour larger than 4 cm in the greatest dimension.

T4a: tumour invades the larynx, deep/extrinsic muscle of tongue, medial pterygoid, hard palate or mandible.

T4b: tumour invades lateral pterygoid muscle, pterygoid plates, lateral nasopharynx, or skull base or encases carotid artery.

v.   As with all head and neck malignancies, this patient would be formally discussed at a multi-disciplinary team (MDT) where a treatment plan would be formulated. Early stage disease (T1–T2) should be treated with a single modality, which may be primary radiotherapy or transoral surgery and neck dissection. The transoral approach is preferred to open surgery and is associated with good functional outcomes. If treated surgically, selective neck dissection involves levels II–IV and possibly level I. If there is no disease evident in level IIa then Level IIb can be omitted. Chemotherapy is not routinely used in early-stage disease.

vi. Occult neck metastases are present in 10%–31% of patients with T1–T2 disease and the treatment of a N0 neck remains a controversial topic. Those undergoing primary surgery can undergo a selective neck dissection and for patients treated with primary radiotherapy, prophylactic treatment of the neck is often advised. Sentinel lymph node biopsy is another option unless cervical access is required at the same time as primary surgery.

These decisions should be discussed at the local MDT and based upon any national guidance, which varies from country to country.

CASE 2

QUESTIONS 2

i. What procedure is being carried out?

ii. Describe the advantages and disadvantages for the different types of tubes that can be used with this procedure.

iii. What are the indications for this procedure?

iv. What are the advantages of tracheostomy compared to endotracheal intubation in the ventilated ITU patient?

v. What are the complications of tracheostomy?

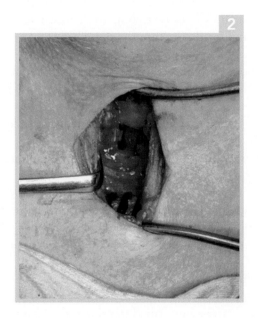

Answers 2

i.   Tracheostomy

ii.   There are a number of tracheostomy tubes available: cuffed tubes (non-fenestrated and fenestrated), uncuffed tubes (non-fenestrated and fenestrated), cuffed adjustable flange tubes and silver negus tubes. The majority of tubes have inner and outer tubes; the inner tube can be easily removed for cleaning without disturbing the outer tube.

Fenestrated tubes enable patients to talk by allowing airflow to pass superiorly through the fenestrations and through the vocal cords. However, there is a risk of aspiration with fenestrated tubes and they should only be used in patients with a safe swallowing mechanism.

Cuffed tubes prevent leaking of secretions around the tube into the lungs and provide an airtight seal to enable positive pressure ventilation. However, prolonged use of a cuff can cause trauma to the tracheal wall: tracheomalacia, tracheal stenosis and fistulation into the oesophagus.

Cuff pressures should be checked regularly using a manometer. Most modern tubes have a high-volume, low-pressure cuff to minimise these risks.

A cuffed adjustable flange can be useful in patients with deep neck.

Silver negus tubes are uncuffed and only used in some long-term tracheostomy patients.

iii. One of the most common reasons to undertake a tracheostomy is to bypass upper airway obstruction. This is usually carried out as an emergency but is occasionally required following head and neck surgery if post-operative oedema is likely.

Patients with bulbar problems often accumulate excessive secretions that put them at risk of aspiration. Tracheostomy followed by insertion of a cuffed tracheostomy tube can be performed to protect the airway. Finally, if a patient on intensive care has been ventilated via an endotracheal tube for a prolonged period of time, the endotracheal tube can be replaced with a tracheostomy tube.

iv.   Placement of a tracheostomy tube within the first 14 days of intubation reduces the risk of tracheal trauma with subsequent stenosis. It also reduces the amount of dead space in the respiratory system and the effort of breathing. This makes weaning easier. It also reduces the need for sedation and permits speech and oral feeding once the patient is awake.

A tracheostomy tube also makes re-ventilation much easier should it be required.

v. The complications of tracheostomy are:
- Local damage
- Dislodgement
- Infection
- Tracheal necrosis
- Tracheoarterial fistula
- TOF
- Dysphagia
- Tracheal stenosis
- Tracheocutaneous fistula

QUESTIONS 3

A 53-year-old gentleman presented with a slowly growing lesion at the right angle of jaw. Histology following a superficial parotidectomy (see image) showed a Warthins tumour that was completely excised. He presents 2 years following his surgery complaining of sweating on the right side of his face when he eats.

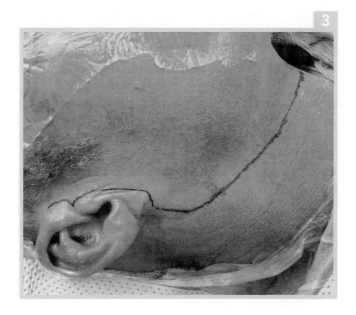

i.   What is the likely diagnosis?

ii. How would you diagnose it?

iii. What are the available treatment options?

Answers 3

i.   Frey's syndrome – This is a post-parotidectomy condition that can develop up
      to several years post-surgery. Aberrant innervation of cutaneous sweat glands
      overlying the parotid gland by postganglionic parasympathetic salivary nerves
      results in localised sweating during eating or salivation. The incidence of Frey
      syndrome varies widely and may correlate with the amount of gland removed
      such that the greater the quantity of parotid tissue removed, the greater the
      amount of raw surface available to provide aberrant innervation to the skin. To
      minimise this risk, it is possible to interpose gland capsule, autologous tissue or
      alloplastic biological material between the gland and the skin.

ii.   Diagnosis is usually based on a characteristic history and clinical findings. The
      Minor iodine–starch test is useful in localising the condition.

iii. Most patients will not pursue treatment due to mild symptoms. If symptoms
      are problematic, however, there are surgical and non-surgical options available.
      Topical anticholinergics and antihydrotics can be used. Botulinum A toxin is also
      a popular but temporary treatment. Surgical options include excision of affected
      areas or the use tissue interposition. These procedures do, however, put the facial
      nerve at significant risk and have limited success. They are therefore infrequently
      used.

CASE 4

A 62-year-old man presents to the emergency department following a fire at his house. The appearance of his nose is shown in the image.

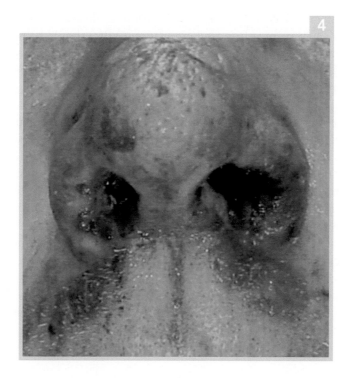

i.   What are the signs and symptoms of smoke inhalation injury?

ii.   How would you manage a patient who presents with an inhalation injury?

iii. When is it necessary to secure the airway after smoke inhalation injury?

i.   Signs of smoke inhalation injury may include facial burns, blistering or oedema
        of the oropharynx, hoarse voice, stridor, carbonaceous sputum, hair singeing,
        tachypnoea, central nervous system depression, coma and cyanosis. Symptoms
        may include dyspnoea, odynophagia, cough, wheezing, irritability, headaches
        and lethargy.

ii.   When a patient presents with smoke inhalation, immediate assessment of
        the patient's airway, breathing and circulation (ABC) should be undertaken.
        Intravenous (IV) access, cardiac monitoring and supplemental oxygen in the
        setting of hypoxia should be provided. Arterial blood gases can be very helpful in
        determining the extent of the inhalation injury.

        Some patients manifest bronchospasm and may benefit from the use of
        bronchodilators. Patients who are at low risk for injury and whose vital signs
        and physical examination findings remain normal can usually be discharged
        after 8–12 hours of monitoring with close follow-up and instructions to return
        if symptoms develop. Those with the following should be admitted to hospital
        and investigated: history of closed-space exposure for longer than 10 min,
        carbonaceous sputum production, arterial PO2 less than 60 mm Hg, metabolic
        acidosis, carboxyhaemoglobin levels above 15%, bronchospasm, odynophagia and
        central facial burns.

iii.   When upper airway injury is suspected or there is evidence of respiratory failure
        and/or declining oxygenation levels, elective intubation should be considered.
        Airway oedema can progress over the next 24–48 hours and may make later
        intubation difficult if not impossible.

QUESTIONS 5

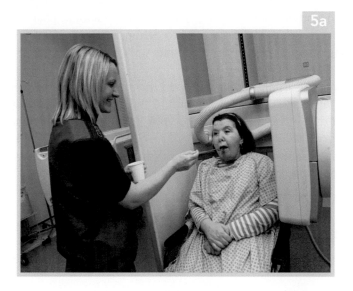

5a

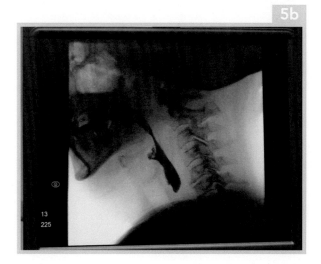

5b

i. What is the procedure being performed in these images?

ii. How is it useful in evaluating swallowing disorders?

i.   Videofluoroscopy

ii.   Videofluoroscopy is essentially a recorded modified barium swallow. It is designed to study the anatomy and physiology of the oral, pharyngeal, and oesophageal stages of deglutition and to define treatment strategies to improve swallowing safety or efficiency in patients with dysphagia.

It allows a frame-by-frame evaluation of the rapid sequence of events involved in transfer of the bolus from the mouth to the oesophagus. It can also document oral motor dysfunction, pharyngeal incoordination, nasopharyngeal reflux, laryngeal penetration or aspiration, gastro-oesophageal reflux and hiatal hernia. The speech therapist can use it to identify means of improving swallow (food texture, consistency and size; patient positioning).

CASE 6

QUESTIONS 6

A 9-year-old child had a tonsillectomy performed 9 days ago for recurrent tonsillitis. He presents to accident and emergency with bleeding from his oropharynx. When you examine him, he is haemodynamically stable and the appearance of his oropharynx is shown as follows. Whilst he is waiting to be transferred to the ward, he begins to bleed again.

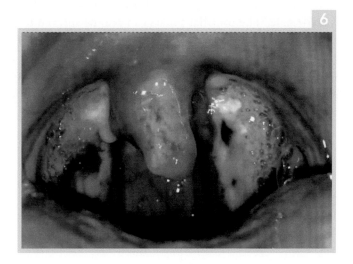

i.   What percentage of blood loss will result in hypotension in a child?

ii.   How do you estimate a child's blood volume?

iii.   How do you calculate the volume for the initial fluid resuscitation?

iv.   What are the common surgical methods used to arrest the bleeding?

i.   20%–25% blood loss.

ii.   The approximate blood volume is 80 mL/kg.

iii.   The child should initially be resuscitated with 20 mL/kg of fluid.

iv.   Arrest of bleeding can be acheived in several ways. If there is a specific bleeding point it can be electrocauterised or tied although the latter is often difficult as the tonsil beds are friable. The tonsillar pillars can also be sutured together. At the end of the procedure, a nasogastric (NG) tube should be passed into the stomach to aspirate any swallowed blood. Very rarely the external carotid artery may have to be ligated. Any blood coagulopathies should be treated appropriately if indicated.

CASE 7

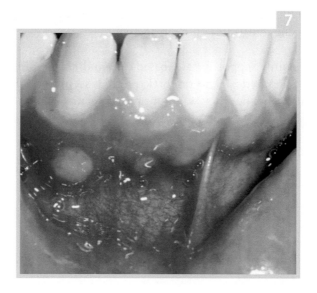

QUESTIONS 7

A 29-year-old man presents with numerous lesions within the oral cavity (see image). They tend to come and go and are painful when present.

i.   What does the image show?

ii.   What are the predisposing factors for this condition?

iii. What are the treatment options?

i.   The image shows aphthous ulcers.

ii.   Predisposing factors include a positive family history, haematinic deficiency (iron, folate, vitamin B), malabsorption in gastrointestinal disorders (Crohn's disease, coeliac disease), stress, cessation of smoking, trauma (biting, dentures), allergies to food (cow milk), drug reaction (non-steroidal anti-inflammatory drugs [NSAIDs], alendronate, nicorandil) and immunodeficiency (human immunodeficiency virus [HIV], neutropenia).

iii.   Treatment is mainly supportive and based on avoiding any predisposing factors. Topical local anaesthetic agents or corticosteroids seem to be the most efficacious in symptomatic relief but they will not prevent recurrence.

CASE 8

A 56-year-old gentleman complains of a rapidly growing lesion on his lower lip. It has doubled in size in the last month. He thinks he may have accidentally bitten his lip prior to the lesion appearing.

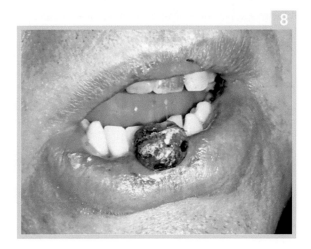

i.   What is the likely diagnosis?

ii.   How would you treat it?

Answers 8

i. The likely diagnosis is a pyogenic granuloma. The name is misleading – it is not associated with pus and does not represent a granuloma histologically. It is a reactive inflammatory process.

ii. This requires surgical excision and confirmation of the diagnosis with histology. The lesion lies on the inner aspect of the lip. It can, therefore, be excised and closed primarily ensuring the lower lip does not become notched. An alternative method would be to excise the lesion and let the area heal by secondary intention.

CASE 9

A 65-year-old gentleman complains of a 2-day history of left jaw pain followed by rapid onset of neck swelling. On examination, he looks unwell and is pyrexial. There is no stridor but he is finding it difficult to talk due to limited mouth opening.

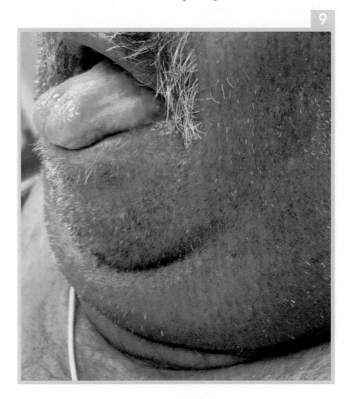

i.   What is the likely diagnosis shown in the picture?

ii.   What is the cause of the condition?

iii. How it is best treated?

i.   This is Ludwig's angina. It is characterised by a rapidly progressive cellulitis of the soft tissues of the neck and floor of the mouth. With progressive swelling of the soft tissues and elevation and posterior displacement of the tongue, the most life-threatening complication of Ludwig's angina is airway obstruction. The submandibular space is the primary site of infection. This space is divided by the mylohyoid muscle into a submaxillary space inferiorly and sublingual space superiorly.

ii.   In 90% of cases the cause is odontogenic in origin, primarily from the second and third molars as their roots penetrate the mylohyoid ridge such that any abscess or dental infection has direct access to the submandibular space, parapharyngeal space and retropharyngeal space, thereby potentially encircling the airway.

Other causes include penetrating injuries and mandibular fractures.

iii.   Airway management is the foundation of treatment for patients with Ludwig's angina. The decision to secure the airway relies on clinical judgment and experience. Intravenous antibiotics (combinations of penicillin, clindamycin and metronidazole are typically used) should be started as soon as possible. Once the airway is deemed to be secure the neck should be imaged. Contrast enhanced computed tomography (CT) is the most frequently used modality and can identify abscess formation that occurs in two thirds of patients. Any abscess should be drained once the airway is secure. The source of the infection (e.g. infected tooth/teeth) should also be addressed.

QUESTIONS 10

This is an image of a 56-year-old gentleman with a 3-week history of a thyroid swelling.

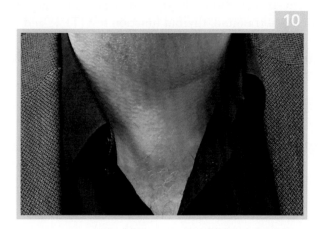

i.   What are the pertinent questions to ask when taking a history?

ii.   What investigations would you request for this patient?

iii.   Are you aware of any cytological grading system for thyroid lesions?

iv.   What types of malignancy can occur in the thyroid gland?

v.   How should a malignancy in the thyroid gland be treated?

i.   The following symptoms should be queried: Pain, dysphagia, voice change, aspiration, breathing difficulties, family history of thyroid cancer, history of radiation exposure and symptoms of hyper/hypothyroidism.

ii. Investigations for lesions within the thyroid gland should be, fine needle aspiration (FNA), ultrasound, thyroid function test (TFT) and thyroid antibodies.

iii. The cytological grading system for thyroid lesions is the Thy classification: This consists of:

Thy1: Non-diagnostic

Thy2: Non-neoplastic

Thy3: Follicular lesion/suspected follicular neoplasm

Thy4: Suspicious of malignancy (suspicious, but not diagnostic, of papillary, medullary or anaplastic carcinoma, or lymphoma)

Thy5: Diagnostic of malignancy (unequivocal features of papillary, medullary or anaplastic carcinoma, lymphoma or metastatic tumour)

iv. There are four types of primary thyroid malignancy: papillary, follicular, medullary and anaplastic carcinoma. The thyroid can also be affected by lymphoma and very occasionally can be the site of metastases.

v.   The treatment of choice for most forms of thyroid malignancy is total thyroidectomy unless the tumour is very small (<1 cm). This may be in combination with central neck dissection +/− lateral neck dissection. Radio-iodine ablation may be used post-operatively if the tumour is greater than 4 cm, if there are known distant metastses, if there is significant extra-thyroid extension or if scintigraphy identifies previously unrecognised disease. All patients receive post-operative thyroxine treatment. In papillary and follicular malignancy, the aim is to reduce thyroid stimulating hormone levels to <0.1 mU/L. This is not as important in medullary carcinomas as the cell of origin (C-cells) are not thyroxine sensitive.

Radiotherapy and chemotherapy are only used for limited indications eg. unresectable tumours. Tyrosine kinase inhibitors are the main chemotherapeutic agents used eg. sorafenib. Anaplastic tumours are very aggressive and are usually advanced at presentation. They are often not amenable to surgery unless they are small. They may be treated chemoradiotherapy.

CASE 11

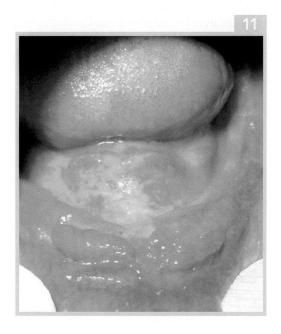

QUESTIONS 11

A 75-year-old man presents to your clinic with a swelling in his mouth. He has been wearing dentures for many years.

i. What is shown in the photograph?

ii. What investigations are needed to diagnose the condition?

iii. What are the treatment options?

Answers 11

i. Epulis fissuratum is mucosal hyperplasia that results from chronic low-grade trauma induced by a denture flange. Epulis is the consequence of resorption of the alveolar ridge so that the denture moves further into the vestibular mucosa, creating an inflammatory fibrous hyperplasia that proliferates over the flange. Patients are usually asymptomatic.

ii. As the differential for Epulis is squamous cell carcinoma, surgical excision (with or without laser) is indicated for diagnostic and therapeutic purposes.

iii. Removal of the offending stimulus, that is the denture, will result in complete resolution.

CASE 12

A 74-year-old patient presented with a 6-month history of a painless lump between the ear lobule and angle of the jaw with no skin changes or recent change in size.

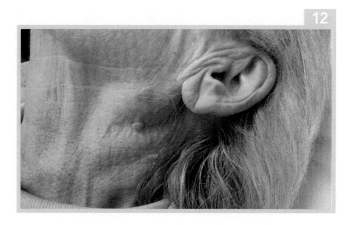

i.   What is the differential diagnosis?

ii. How would you investigate this lump?

iii. What treatment, if any, would you offer the patient?

iv. What consent issues would you discuss with the patient prior to surgery?

i.   Most likely this is a benign parotid tumour. As 80% of benign parotid tumours are pleomorphic salivary adenomas (PSAs), this would be the most likely diagnosis. Other possible diagnoses include other benign parotid tumours such as Warthin's (adenolymphoma) tumour, intra-/extra-parotid lymph node, malignant mass, metastasis or haemangioma.

ii.   The most useful investigation is fine-needle aspiration cytology with overall accuracy greater than 96%. Imaging with either ultrasound scanning or magnetic resonance imaging (MRI) scans is complementary but not essential in benign disease and is reserved for patients with any 'red flag' symptoms such as a recent increase in size, skin involvement, fixed hard mass and/or facial nerve weakness.

iii. If cytology reveals the diagnosis of PSA, a partial superficial parotidectomy is usually offered to the patient depending on their fitness for a general anaesthetic. The patient should be counselled about the fact that PSA has a 2%–10% chance of malignant transformation if observed for a long period.

iv.   Consent discussion should mention the risk of temporary/permanent injury to the facial nerve quoting percentages from each specific surgical unit. Numbness to the ear lobule, scarring and soft-tissue defect, salivary fistula, seroma, infection, Frey syndrome and recurrence should also be discussed with the patient. Enucleation, apart from selected cases of Warthin's tumours or lymph nodes, is not indicated for PSA surgery.

QUESTIONS 13

A 57-year-old male electrician is referred with a 3-month history of worsening dysphonia. Co-morbidities include hypertension. He has smoked 30 cigarettes per day for 40 years and drinks 40 units of alcohol per week. Flexible nasendoscopy reveals a lesion on the left vocal cord. Cord mobility is normal. There are no neck nodes palpable. Direct laryngoscopy at the time of biopsy is shown as follows.

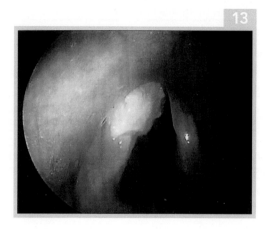

i.   What is the diagnosis?

ii. What is the most common subsite for this pathology?

iii. Outline the 'T' classification (of the TNM) for this subsite.

iv. What are the treatment options for a T1 lesion of this subsite? Outline the benefits of each approach.

i. There is an exophytic, keratotic lesion on the left vocal cord. The most likely diagnosis is squamous cell carcinoma of the larynx.

ii. The glottis is the most common subsite, accounting for 50% of tumours. Forty percent arise in the supraglottis and 10% in the subglottis.

iii. The T classification for carcinoma of the glottis is:

a.

T1	Tumour limited to the vocal cord(s) (may involve anterior or posterior commissure) with normal mobility
T1a	Tumour limited to one vocal cord
T1b	Tumour involves both vocal cords
T2	Tumour extends to supraglottis and/or subglottis, and/or with impaired vocal cord mobility
T3	Tumour limited to the larynx with vocal cord fixation and/or invades paraglottic space, and/or minor thyroid cartilage erosion (e.g. inner cortex)
T4a	Tumour invades through the thyroid cartilage and/or invades tissues beyond the larynx (e.g. trachea, soft tissues of the neck including deep extrinsic muscles of the tongue, strap muscles, thyroid or esophagus)
T4b	Tumour invades prevertebral space, encases carotid artery or invades mediastinal structures

iv. Early laryngeal malignancy is usually treated with single modality therapy. The options are as follows:
- Radiotherapy.
  Transoral laser microsurgery.
- Transoral robotic surgery is performed in some centres.
  At present there is insufficient evidence to suggest any one modality is superior in terms of local control or survival rates. Surgical resection without the use of the laser has declined over the past decade.
  Transoral laser microsurgery is now the mainstay of surgical treatment and the research suggests that it is associated with higher rates of long term laryngeal preservation when compared to radiotherapy. There is debate about which modality provides superior voice function. Proponents of radiotherapy state that voice function is better with this modality but equally some studies have shown comparable or superior outcomes with transoral laser and this remains a contentious issue. The side effects of radiotherapy can be significant and, in cases of recurrent disease, it increases the morbidity of salvage surgery. As with all head and neck malignancies, the case should be discussed at a multi-disciplinary team (MDT) meeting to ensure the appropriate treatment for each patient.

QUESTIONS 14

A 57-year-old woman is 2 days post left modified radical neck dissection (type 3). Routine review reveals a drainage output of 700 mL/24 h and the drain contents have a creamy, white appearance.

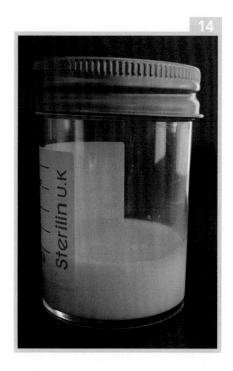

i.   What is the likely diagnosis?

ii.   How would this be confirmed?

iii.   How can this be classified?

iv.   Outline the conservative management strategy of this complication (including medical therapy).

v.   When is surgical intervention usually considered? What surgical procedures are used in the management?

Answers 14

i. This is a chyle leak. It is caused by intra-operative injury to the thoracic duct. The drain output and creamy white appearance are characteristic. This complication is usually detected post-operatively by unexpectedly high drain output, sudden increase in drain output when resuming/establishing oral intake with creamy, or 'milky tea' coloured fluid in the drain bottle or tubing.

ii. A drain fluid sample can be sent for triglyceride analysis. Triglyceride levels of >100 mg/dL or a level greater than that of serum are diagnostic.

iii. Leaks are classified according to output, although there is some variation as to what constitutes high and low output. Generally,

Low output < 500 mL/24 h

High output >1 L/24 h

There is variation as to how outputs of >500 mL but <1 L are classified, with some regarding them as low and others intermediate.

iv. Conservative therapy is indicated for low-output leaks. Key components include the following:
- Bed rest.
- Leave drain in situ.
- Nutrition: a modified fat-free or medium-chain triglyceride diet can be delivered enterally. Total parenteral nutrition is widely used but there is no consensus as to the most appropriate timing. Some advocate immediate use, whereas others recommend use in leaks persisting beyond 3–5 days.
- Medical therapies, such as Octreotide and Orlistat, have been trialed to inhibit chyle production but have not proven to be of significant benefit and evidence is limited to small case series.
- Skin care: chyle is extremely irritant to skin and surrounding tissues; tissue care is paramount to prevent wound breakdown.
- Electrolyte monitoring: high-output leaks can cause severe electrolyte imbalances. Electrolytes should be monitored closely and problems treated early.
- If the drainage is impeded, sepsis can ensue and washout with re-establishment of drainage and antibiotic therapy will be required.
- If repeated aspirations are attempted then clinicians should be vigilant for septic complications.

v.   Surgery can be classified into local and distal procedures.

Local: involves re-exploration of the neck with a view to ligation of the leak site. Coverage of the leak area with a local muscle flap is advocated by some. Local surgery to the neck is only usually indicated in the first 24 hours as, beyond that, the tissues have been subject to extensive chylous contamination, leading to a florid inflammatory reaction.

Distal:
- Thoracic duct embolisation.
- Endoscopic/thorascopic ligation of the thoracic duct (VATS). Referral to the cardiothoracic surgeons for video-assisted thoracoscopic surgery is appropriate for high-output leaks or low-output ones that fail to respond to conservative management.

CASE 15

QUESTIONS 15

A 67-year-old gentleman presents with multiple malignant neck nodes arising from a tonsillar carcinoma.

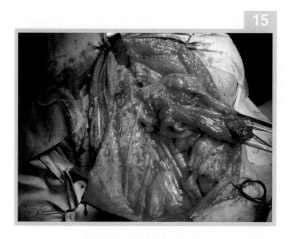

i.   What procedure is being carried out in the picture?

ii.   How is this procedure classified?

iii. What are the complications of this procedure?

iv.   How is neck disease staged (N) in the TNM classification system with respect to the upper aerodigestive tract (excluding nasopharyngeal carcinoma)?

i.   The procedure being performed is a neck dissection.

ii.   These are broadly classified into the following:
   - Radical
   - Modified radical
   - Selective
   - Extended radical

Selective neck dissections preserve one or more lymph node levels and at least one or all of the following: internal jugular vein (IJV), accessory nerve (CN XI) and sternocleidomastoid muscle (SCM). Their purpose is to resect the lymph node groups deemed to have the highest risk of metastases and preserve all non-lymphatic structures. Different types of selective neck disection include:
   - Supra-omohyoid (Levels I–III)
     - Lip and oral cavity malignancy
   - Lateral (Levels II–IV)
     - Laryngeal and hypopharyngeal malignancy
   - Posterolateral (Levels II–V)
     - Skin malignancy
   - Anterior compartment (Levels VI $\pm$ VII)
     - Thyroid and some laryngeal malignancies

Modified radical neck dissections are classified as type 1, 2 and 3, according to the non-lymphatic structures preserved. Levels I–V are removed.
   - Type 1: preservation of CN XI
   - Type 2: preservation of CN XI and IJV
   - Type 3: preservation of CN XI, IJV and SCM. This was previously referred to as a functional neck dissection.

A radical neck dissection involves removal of the following:
   - Lymph node levels I–V
   - IJV
   - CN XI
   - SCM
   - Submandibular gland

The procedure can be classed as an extended radical neck dissection if further lymph node levels or another non-nodal structure are removed.

iii.   Complications include the following:

Early:
- Haemorrhage
- Infection
- Skin flap necrosis
- Nerve injury: CNX, XI, marginal mandibular, lingual, sympathetic trunk
- Chlye leak and chylous fistula
- Facial oedema: increased risk with IJV ligation
- Cerebral oedema: increased risk with IJV ligation
- Carotid artery rupture: usually associated with wound breakdown or previous radiotherapy

Late:
- Recurrence: nodal or skin incision
- Chronic neck/shoulder pain
- Carotid artery rupture

iv.   **Nx:** regional nodes cannot be assessed

N0: no regional lymph node metastasis

N1: metastasis in a single ipsilateral lymph node 3 cm or less in greatest dimension

N2a: metastasis in a single ipsilateral lymph node >3 cm but <6 cm in greatest dimension

N2b: metastasis in multiple ipsilateral lymph nodes <6 cm in greatest dimension

N2c: metastasis in bilateral or contralateral lymph nodes <6 cm in greatest dimension

N3: metastasis to any lymph node more than 6 cm in greatest dimension

CASE 16

QUESTIONS 16

A 19-year-old woman presents with a 3-day history of sore throat, fever and dysphagia. On examination she is noted to have a muffled voice, marked trismus and drooling. The right tonsil is displaced medially and there is some swelling and induration at the angle of the mandible.

A contrast computed tomography (CT) neck is shown in the image.

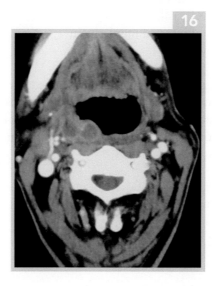

i.   What is the most likely diagnosis?

ii.   What are the most likely sources of infection?

iii. What are the complications?

iv.   What are the boundaries of this anatomical space and what are the contents?

v.   How would you manage this patient?

i. The diagnosis is a parapharyngeal abscess. The history and examination findings are typical of this and the diagnosis is confirmed on CT.

ii. Typical infection sources are tonsils, pharynx, nasopharynx, parotid and teeth.

iii. Complications include the following:
- Airway obstruction
- Spread to adjacent deep neck spaces eg. retropharyngeal and carotid spaces, which then permits extension to mediastinum
- Cranial nerve IX–XI palsies
- Thrombophlebitis of internal jugular vein
- Carotid artery blowout

iv. The parapharyngeal space is shaped like an inverted pyramid, with the skull base superiorly (i.e. the base) and the hyoid bone inferiorly (at the apex). It is bound posteriorly by prevertebral fascia and laterally the medial pterygoids, mandible and deep lobe of parotid. Medially it is bound by the buccopharyngeal fascia overlying the pharyngeal constrictors.

A fascial condensation from the styloid process to the tensor veli palatini muscle divides the space into pre- and post-styloid compartments.

The pre-styloid compartment contains the following:
- Maxillary artery
- Fat
- Inferior alveolar/lingual/auriculotemporal nerves
- Deep lobe of the parotid gland
- Lymph nodes

The post-styloid compartment contains the following:
- Carotid artery
- Internal jugular vein
- Cranial nerves IX, X, XI
- Sympathetic chain
- Lymph nodes

v. In the clinically stable patient, with a small abscess, with no evidence of complications, medical treatment with intravenous (IV) antibiotics is the first line of treatment. It is important to ensure that the antibiotics used cover gram-positive cocci and anaerobes. The most commonly identified aerobes are Group A *Streptococcus*, *Prevotella*, *Fusobacterium* and *Haemophilus influenzae* (although this can grow as a facultative anaerobe). The most common anaerobes are *Staphylococcus aureus* and *Peptostreptococcus*.

If patients respond well to IV antibiotics then this medical approach can be continued. However, if they fail to respond or worsen, surgical incision and drainage are required. Surgery is also considered as first line in those presenting with complications or a large collection. A transcervical approach is used, making a transverse incision at the level of the greater cornu of the hyoid about two-finger breadth below the angle of the mandible.

QUESTIONS 17

A 50-year-old woman is referred to you from the endocrine team with a 1-year history of lethargy and headaches. Blood investigations reveal hypercalcaemia and, as part of her investigations, the following imaging is obtained.

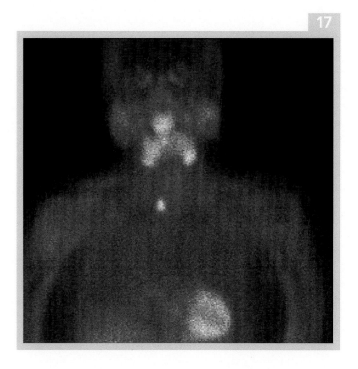

i.   Which investigation is shown and what is the most likely diagnosis?

ii.   Which other radiological investigation is routinely performed pre-operatively to aid localisation?

iii.   If both these radiological investigations are negative, what other investigations can be performed?

Answers 17

i. This is a scintigraph using Technicium99 indicating a right lower parathyroid adenoma. Used alone this scan will detect 87% of solitary adenomas. In patients with multiple gland disease, only 55% of abnormal glands will be identified.

ii. Ultrasound is commonly used in conjunction with a Sestamibi scan. With an experienced radiologist, sensitivity and specificity can reach 96% and 100%, respectively.

iii. Computed tomography (CT) can be useful for detection of ectopic glands.

Magnetic resonance imaging (MRI) can be useful for detection of ectopic glands and should be considered in previous failed parathyroidectomy.

Positron emission tomography–computed tomography (PET-CT) will detect 88% of adenomas.

CASE 18

A 21-year-old man is brought to the emergency department having sustained a penetrating neck injury.

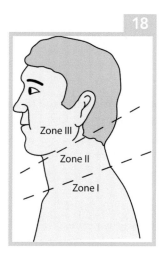

i.   To what do the different zones above refer?

ii.   What are the indications for mandatory neck exploration following penetrating neck trauma?

iii.   Outline the management of the following clinical scenarios:

     a.   A 25-year-old man, Zone II injury with dysphagia, odynophagia and voice change. Haemodynamically stable.

     b.   A 19-year-old man, Zone I injury with dysphagia and surgical emphysema. Haemodynamically stable.

     c.   Zone I injury, haemodynamically unstable, large wound with air blowing through.

     d.   Zone III injury, haemodynamically unstable, expanding haematoma.

iv.   What is the most commonly missed injury in penetrating neck injury?

Answers 18

i. Roon and Christensen's classification divides the anterior neck into three zones:

Zone I. Sternal notch to cricoid cartilage. At-risk structures are the following:
- Proximal common carotid arteries
- Vertebral and subclavian arteries
- Subclavian, innominate and jugular veins
- Trachea
- Recurrent laryngeal and vagus nerves
- Oesophagus
- Thoracic duct

Zone II. This extends from cricoid cartilage to angle of mandible. In this zone the at-risk structures are as follows:
- Carotid sheath
- Internal jugular and vertebral veins
- Pharynx
- Larynx
- Proximal trachea
- Recurrent laryngeal and vagus nerves
- Spinal cord

Zone III. Angle of mandible to skull base.
- Distal carotid and vertebral arteries
- Parotid
- Pharynx
- Jugular veins
- Spinal cord
- Cranial nerves IX–XII
- Cranial nerve VII
- Sympathetic trunk

ii. Management of penetrating trauma is much debated and there are currently no UK guidelines. Much of the guidance is derived from the United States and South Africa, but the United Kingdom has much lower rates and different patterns of trauma. It is generally agreed that mandatory neck exploration and panendoscopy is required for the following:
- Airway compromise
- Expanding haematoma
- Haemodynamic instability – not responsive to resuscitation
- Haemoptysis
- Air escaping through wound

iii. a. This is suggestive of a pharyngeal injury. In a stable patient, diagnostic studies can be performed, involving a contrast swallow and CT angiography neck, prior to any surgery. A panendoscopy would then be performed. Conservative versus surgical management is debated. Generally, large perforations below the level of the arytenoids require repair. Small lacerations with no tissue loss above the level of the arytenoids can be considered for conservative management. Antibiotic prophylaxis is indicated and a period of enteral or parenteral nutrition required.

   b. Likely oesophageal injury. In a stable patient, diagnostic studies can be performed, involving a contrast swallow and CT neck/thorax, prior to any surgery. A panendoscopy and/or flexible endoscopy would then be performed. Management of perforations usually requires surgical repair. However, conservative treatment can be considered in patients with small, self-contained perforations and no evidence of complications. Antibiotic prophylaxis is indicated and a period of enteral or parenteral nutrition required.

   Note that oesophageal injuries are associated with higher incidence of airway injury.

   c. Tracheal injury. The first priority is to ensure a secure airway. Surgical exploration and repair is indicated. This may require cardiothoracic involvement. The patient is also haemodynamically unstable and there may be vascular injury. Exploration of the great vessels is also important.

   d. Carotid artery injury. Urgent surgical exploration is required in this case in order to repair the vascular injury.

iv. Oesophageal injuries are most commonly missed, up to 25% patients will be asymptomatic.

CASE 19

QUESTIONS 19

A 56-year-old woman presents with a history of gradual dysphagia over the last 18 months with episodes of regurgitation. You organise the following investigation:

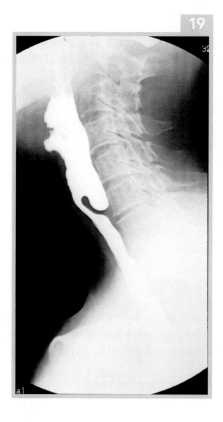

i. What investigation is shown?

ii. What is the diagnosis and aetiology?

iii. What symptoms and signs might the patient present with?

iv. What are the treatment options?

v. Is there a risk of malignancy?

i. Barium swallow.

ii. Pharyngeal pouch, also known as a Zenker diverticulum. These are pulsion diverticula of the oesophageal mucosa that prolapse through the posterior wall of the oesophagus at a point of weakness called Killian's dehiscance. This describes an area bound by the horizontal fibres of cricopharyngeus inferiorly and oblique fibres of thyropharyngeus superiorly. The pathophysiology of pharyngeal pouches is unclear but is likley to result from disorder of the cricopharyngeus muscle, whether that be muscular spasm, elevated resting tone, loss of muscle elasticity, myopathy or denervation.

iii. Classical symptoms include the following:
- Food sticking in the throat
- Progressive dysphagia
- Regurgitation of undigested food. This is often exacerbated by change in position such as lying flat
- Halitosis
- Gurgling from the neck
- Weight loss
- Aspiration which may result in pneumonia
- Hoarseness

Signs include the following:
- Neck swelling, usually in the lower left anterior triangle
- Boyce's sign – gurgling on auscultation of the swelling
- Coughing on applying pressure to the swelling – due to aspiration of the contents.

iv. Treatment options include the following:
- Conservative: if asymptomatic/unfit for surgery/declines treatment.
- Endoscopic dilatation – this dilates the cricopharyngeal sphincter for temporary relief but does not address the underlying pathology.
- Endoscopic stapling: divides the bar between the pouch and oesophagus, thus widening the mouth of the pouch to facilitate swallowing. This is the procedure of choice with shorter in-patient stay and lower morbidity.
- Open procedure/external approach: the pouch may be excised (diverticulectomy), inverted or suspended. This approach is less common now and is usually reserved for pouches that are not accessible endoscopically or that have recurred.

v. There is a possibility of carcinoma occurring within a pouch, first described in 1927 by Vinson. However, it is rare with a risk of 0.4%.

CASE 20

QUESTIONS 20

A 50-year-old man presents to your clinic complaining of white discoloration within his mouth. He has a history of moderate consumption of alcohol and cigarettes.

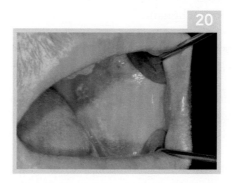

i.   What is the differential diagnosis?

ii. What investigations are needed?

iii. What treatment options are available?

i.   This clinical photograph shows white striation over the left buccal mucosa, which most likely represents oral lichen planus (OLP). OLP can present as white striations (Wickham striae), white papules, white plaques, erythema (mucosal atrophy), erosions (shallow ulcers) or blisters. The lesions predominantly affect the buccal mucosa, tongue and gingivae, although other oral sites are occasionally involved. The lesions are usually bilateral and are considered, controversially, pre-malignant.

Differential diagnosis includes oral leukoplakia, oral dysplasia (carcinoma *in situ*), candidiasis, dermatitis, graft versus host disease and autoimmune blistering diseases.

ii.   A biopsy is essential to rule out malignant disease as just fewer than 5% of OLP can transform into squamous cell carcinoma. Skin patch testing may be helpful in identifying a contact allergy in some patients with OLP.

iii.   The aims of treatment are resolution of painful symptoms, resolution of oral ulceration, minimising the risk of recurrence and of malignant transformation. It is often not possible to completely resolve OLP and an acceptable end point of treatment is stable asymptomatic striations or papules.

Treatments include:

1.   Good oral hygiene, including maintenance of dentition and adequately fitting prostheses.

2.   Avoidance of any pre-disposing drugs if possible eg. NSAIDs, Beta blockers.

3.   Avoidance of risk factors for oral cancer eg. smoking and excessive alcohol consumption.

4.   Use of topical steroids to stabilise erosive, symptomatic lesions.

CASE 21

QUESTIONS 21

A 5-year-old child presents with a history of recurrent swelling in their mouth. On examination you find the following.

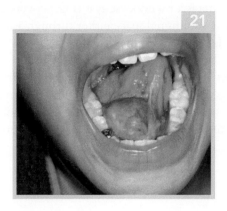

i.   Describe the condition in this picture?

ii.   How does this condition develop?

iii. What is the best treatment option?

i.   This is a clinical picture of a young patient showing a cystic swelling in the right floor of the mouth. This is a ranula.

ii.   A ranula represents a cystic extravasation mucocele that arises from the sublingual gland usually after a torn duct of rivinus or ruptured acini due to obstruction. A ranula is a pseudocyst as it is not covered by epithelium. Ranulae can plunge into the sublingual space either through a mylohyoid hiatus or around the posterior border of the mylohyoid muscle.

iii.   Treatment options are numerous and include simple drainage, injecting the cyst with sclerosing agents and marsupalisation. The recurrence rate is high, however, and the most reliable option is excision of the ranula together with the sublingual gland. The reported recurrence rate with this procedure is less than 2%.

QUESTIONS 22

A 50-year-old man presented with recurrent swelling below his left jaw. It is particularly painful around meal times. A computed tomography (CT) scan is shown.

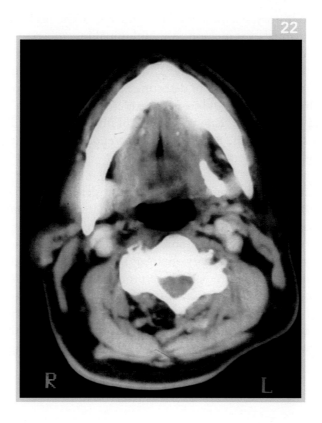

i.   What is the most likely diagnosis?

ii.   How would you manage this patient?

iii. Which nerves are at risk if surgery is undertaken and how would you prevent damage to them?

i. An intraglandular or ductal submandibular stone is the most likely diagnosis. Chronic sialadenitis has a similar presentation with no evidence of stone formation. Other differentials include dental conditions, autoimmune conditions such as Sjögren syndrome, and inflammatory/infective conditions such as sarcoidosis or human immunodeficiency virus (HIV).

ii. After detailed history, examine the lump, the rest of the neck, the oral cavity and perform a bimanual examination. A useful initial investigation is routine plain radiography consisting of intraoral occlusal radiographs, as 70% of submandibular stones are radio-opaque. Ultrasound scans are also very useful in detecting stones, with the added benefit of detecting any solid/cystic lesions and abscess formation. Initially you would treat this patient with hydration, compression, massage and antibiotics if there is evidence of infection in the gland. This will be followed by surgery in the form of radiologic/endoscopic cannulation with stone removal or gland excision in recurrent cases.

iii. The nerves at risk from submandibular gland surgery are the marginal mandibular branch of the facial nerve, the hypoglossal nerve and the lingual nerve. Manoeuvres that aid in preservation of the marginal mandibular nerve include a cervical skin crease incision two-finger breadth inferior to the mandible, a sub-platysmal dissection, ligating the inferior aspect of the posterior facial vein and reflecting it superiorly to protect the marginal mandibular nerve, which lies superior to the vein and inferior to platysma (the Hayes–Martin manoeuvre). Identifying the digastric muscle will guide the surgeon to the hypoglossal nerve thus protecting it, whilst dissecting close to the gland with anterior retraction of the mylohyoid muscle will protect the lingual nerve.

CASE 23

A 20-year-old woman presented to clinic with a history of recurrent infections of a midline neck swelling. Clinically, the swelling moved with tongue protrusion.

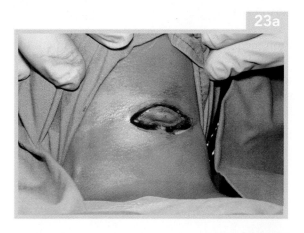

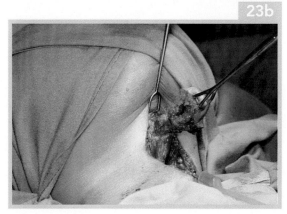

i.   What procedure is being performed in these pictures?

ii.   What is the embryological basis of this condition?

iii. Why does this lesion move on tongue protrusion and swallowing?

iv.   How is the recurrence rate of this surgery minimised?

Answers 23

i.   This is a thyroglossal cyst excision.

ii.   The thyroglossal duct cyst results from the incomplete obliteration of remnants of an epithelial tract formed during migration of the thyroid gland from the foramen cecum in the base of tongue to its final resting position anterior to the trachea in the lower neck.

iii. It moves with tongue protrusion because of its attachment to the hyoid bone.

iv.   Wide local excision of the thyroglossal duct cyst and tract along with a cuff of the tongue base and mid–portion of the hyoid bone will minimise the risk of recurrence.

CASE 24

This is a clinical photograph of a 40-year-old male patient who has been having recurrent tonsillitis for the last few years.

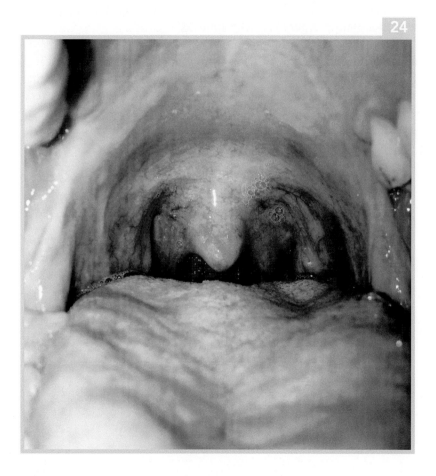

i.   What are the common indications for tonsillectomy?

ii. What are the risks of tonsillectomy?

iii. What is the blood supply to the tonsil?

i. Tonsillectomy is performed for sleep-disordered breathing/obstructive sleep apnoea, recurrent tonsillitis, peritonsillar abscess and tonsils requiring biopsy to define tissue pathology, for example, suspected neoplasm. Less common indications are orthodontic concerns, tonsiliths and halitosis.

ii. Risks include primary and secondary haemorrhage, excessive pain, dental or temporomandibular joint injury, infection, taste distortion and pulmonary oedema (following surgery for sleep apnoea).

iii. The blood supply to the tonsil arises from branches of the external carotid artery. The inferior pole is supplied by the tonsillar branch of the dorsal lingual artery, the tonsillar branch of the facial artery and the ascending palatine artery. The superior pole is supplied by the tonsillar branch of the ascending pharyngeal artery and the lesser palatine artery.

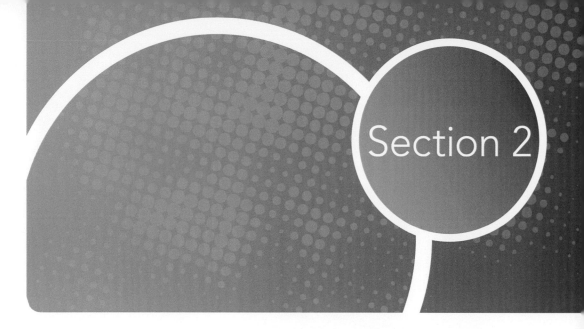

Section 2

LARYNGOLOGY

QUESTIONS 25

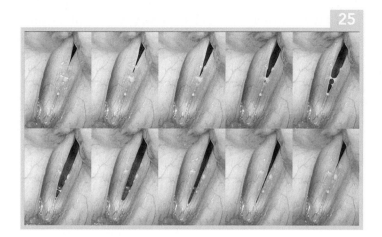

i.   What procedure is shown in these images?

ii.   How does this work?

iii. What are the advantages of using this procedure in evaluating voice disorders?

Answers 25

i.   Stroboscopy.

ii. This is a method of imaging movements of the vocal folds that allows identification of subtle abnormalities of the vocal fold that would otherwise be very difficult to visualise. The vocal folds vibrate when talking but the waves produced in the fold during this process are too rapid to see with the naked eye. Stroboscopy uses a light (the strobe), delivered via a rigid or flexible endoscope, that flashes at a slightly slower speed than the mucosal wave of the vocal fold. This gives the illusion that vocal fold motion is slowed down and makes it much easier to assess vocal fold mobility and the presence of vocal fold pathology.

iii. The main advantages of this technique are the ability to slow down movements of the vocal folds so that pathology can be more easily identified and recording of such abnormalities can be allowed. The main parameters recorded are:

1. The degree of glottic closure

2. Symmetry of vocal fold movement

3. The fundamental frequency of the mucosal wave during vocal fold movement

4. The periodicity of the mucosal wave ie. regularity of the vocal fold wave cycles

5. The amplitude of the mucosal wave

6. The quality of the wave form ie. the organization

QUESTIONS 26

A 60-year-old male smoker presents with a hoarse breathy voice for 4 weeks. Initial endoscopic examination shows the following images.

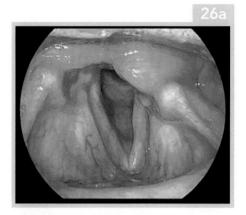

Vocal cord abduction (Courtesy of Dr. Julina Ongkasuwan)

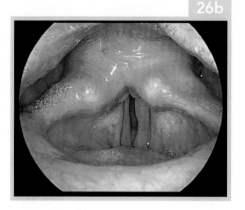

Vocal cord adduction (Courtesy of Dr. Julina Ongkasuwan)

i.   What do the images show?

ii.   What is the next best investigation to perform?

iii. What are the common causes of this condition?

iv.   What are the treatment options and when are they best performed?

i. A left vocal cord palsy.

ii. A computed tomography (CT) scan from base of skull to diaphragm in order
     not to miss any pathology along the course of the vagus and recurrent laryngeal
     nerve (RLN). The course of the left RLN is much longer than the right RLN.
     The right sided RLN leaves the vagus nerve at the root of the neck whereas the
     left RLN leaves the vagus nerve in the chest cavity and then loops around the
     arch of the aorta before travelling back up to the neck.

iii. Iatrogenic injury is the most common cause (either as a result of neck, especially
      thyroid, surgery or cardiothoracic surgery) followed by malignant invasion or
      metastasis from lung, thyroid or head and neck tumours. Vocal cord palsy can
      also be attributed to post-viral illness, neurological diseases (including stroke,
      Parkinson's disease, multiple sclerosis and motor neurone disease) and blunt
      trauma but, in a certain percentage of patients, it is idiopathic.

iv. Treatment should be determined based on the patient's functional needs and
     demands. Treatment usually starts with voice therapy to educate patients on
     proper compensation techniques. Surgical intervention may involve vocal fold
     injection, medialisation thyroplasty or re-innervation surgery. It was considered
     good practice to adopt a watch and wait policy in the first 6 months in case
     spontaneous cord function returns, but there is reasonable evidence now in
     support of early temporary cord injection, which demonstrates better long-term
     voice outcomes.

CASE 27

QUESTIONS 27

A 50-year-old smoker attends clinic with a 3-month history of intermittent hoarse voice. Nasendoscopy findings are as follows:

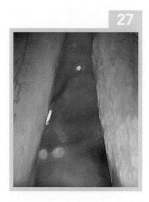

i.   What does it show and what is the likely diagnosis?

ii.   Define this condition and how is it classified?

iii. How do you manage this condition?

iv.   What is the risk of malignant transformation?

i.   This is an endoscopic view of the larynx showing white plaques on the right vocal fold. The likely diagnosis is dysplasia, which will need to be confirmed by biopsy.

ii. Dysplasia is defined as abnormal dyskaryotic squamous cells with cytological alteration including cell shape, size, colour and organisation. It can be classified as follows:
   - Mild: cytological and architectural atypia confined to the basal/parabasal layer
   - Moderate: atypical changes progressing into the mid-spinous layer
   - Severe: progresses into the upper spinous layer

   Carcinoma *in situ* is characterised by atypical changes from basal to spinous layer. The cells demonstrate cytological features of malignancy without invasion of the basement membrane. Severe dysplasia is regarded as synonymous with carcinoma *in situ* and is treated as such. This is a widely accepted premise.

iii. There is debate about the ideal management of laryngeal dysplasia and follow-up period. Useful guidance is provided by ENT-UK. Patients should be stratified into high- and low-risk categories as follows:
   - Low risk
     - Patients who have mild or moderate dysplasia with no visible lesion or hoarseness, or who are not smoking
   - High risk
     - Patients with severe dysplasia or carcinoma *in situ*
     - Patients with mild or moderate dysplasia with one or more of the following:
       - Continued smoking
       - Persistent hoarseness
       - A lesion visible on endoscopy

   For those being managed conservatively, it is recommended that follow-up involves the following:
   - A flexible nasendoscopy to view the larynx
   - Colour photo-documentation retained in the notes
   - Stroboscopy is helpful but not essential

   Low-risk lesions can be followed up by general ENT surgeons in peripheral clinics.

   High-risk lesions should be followed up by a designated ENT surgeon with a special interest in head and neck surgery and/or laryngology.

There are three main ways of managing laryngeal dysplasia: conservative management with careful follow up, surgery aiming to completely excise disease or radiotherapy. Most of the literature suggests no difference in outcome between these groups and in many centres dysplasia is managed conservatively. There is, however, a trend towards active out patient management of this condition with endoscopic laser of the dysplasia increasing in popularity in some centres.

Duration of follow-up

- High-risk patients should be followed up in the same manner as T1 laryngeal carcinoma: monthly for the first year, two monthly for the second year, three monthly in the third year and six monthly in years 4 and 5.
- Low-risk patients should be followed up for a minimum of 6 months. Following that, if the patient agrees, then they may be discharged with instructions to return if there is a change in voice or other suspicious symptoms appear.

iv. There is considerable variation in the literature regarding this figure. Meta-analysis places the overall risk of malignant transformation as 14%. Mild–moderate dysplasia carries a risk of ~10%, rising to 30% with severe dysplasia. There is little evidence at present that indicates the period over which this occurs and the grade does not appear to correlate with time span.

CASE 28

A 40-year-old man attends clinic complaining of a pain in his throat and his left ear. On examination, you see the following image.

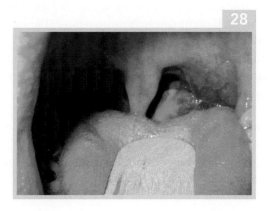

i. What does this show and what is the likely diagnosis?

ii. Which virus is associated with this condition and what is its prognostic significance?

i. There is an exophytic mass arising on the left tonsil, which is highly suspicious for squamous cell carcinoma (SCC).

ii. Human papillomavirus (HPV) type 16 is responsible for the vast majority of HPV-associated SCC. A small number of cases will be HPV type 18 positive.

The oropharynx, lingual and palatine tonsils are the most common sites of HPV-associated SCC. Recent research estimates a 60%–70% prevalence in oropharyngeal SCC. Other subsites have a far lower prevalence, including 24% in the larynx and 21% in the oral cavity. It is also implicated in 25%–50% of unknown primaries, with the presence of HPV in cervical metastases strongly predictive of an oropharyngeal origin.

HPV-positive patients are younger, on average 4–10 years, than non-HPV patients. The overwhelming majority are Caucasian and of higher socioeconomic status. It is more common in men, with HPV type 16 infection being seven times more common. The impact of smoking and alcohol use on HPV-associated SCC is unclear at present.

HPV seems to confer a favourable impact on prognosis but this is tempered by smoking status. Generally, patients present with smaller T staging but more advanced N staging. Overall survival is improved, with 3-year rates of 82% versus 57.1% in non-HPV SCC. A 58% reduction in the risk of death has been demonstrated. Overall, outcomes are best for those that are HPV positive and have never smoked. Those that are HPV positive smokers and those that are HPV negative life-long non-smokers have the next best, and similar prognoses. HPV negative smokers have the worst prognosis.

CASE 29

A 52-year-old woman presents with a 2-month history of a hoarse voice. Nasendoscopy shows the following image.

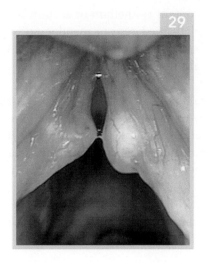

i.   What does the image show?

ii.   Name the two subtypes of pathology that can occur in this condition.

iii.   Name the layers covering the vocal fold.

iv.   How would you excise this lesion?

Answers 29

i. A vocal cord cyst.

ii. Two types of cysts, both of which occur in Reinke's space:
- Mucus retention cysts are often translucent and are lined with cuboidal or columnar epithelium.
- Epidermoid cysts contain epithelium or accumulated keratin. These lesions may be true epithelial-lined cysts or pseudocysts. The term intracordal refers to a location just below the cover of the vocal fold within Reinke space and outside of the vocalis muscle.

iii. The layers of the vocal fold (true vocal cord) consist of a stratified squamous epithelium that covers the superficial, intermediate and deep lamina propria, which themselves overlie the vocalis muscle (thyroarytenoid). Reinke's space is between the epithelium and superficial lamina propria, whilst the intermediate and deep lamina propria layers form the vocal ligament.

iv. Microlaryngoscopic excision is preferable through the microflap approach in order to preserve the mucosal cover with minimal disruption of the underlying tissue.

CASE 30

A 12-year-old girl presents with a history of a 'rough' voice and occasional 'noisy breathing'. Nasendoscopy shows the following image.

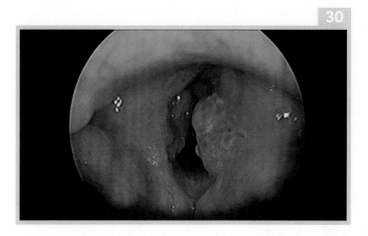

i. What does this show and what is its aetiology?

ii. At what age do they typically occur?

iii. What treatment modalities are used and what are their relative advantages and disadvantages?

iv. What vaccinations may help in the future?

i.   The picture shows laryngeal papillomas. They result from infection with human papilloma virus (HPV) type 6 and type 11 (more aggressive).

ii.   They typically present from the age of 3 years up to early adulthood. The earlier the presentation the more likely it is to be aggressive disease.

iii.   The aims of treatments are to debulk the disease to maintain a good airway and voice without causing significant scarring. The papillomas tend to recur at their original site but may progress with new lesions developing in adjacent laryngeal tissues. In more severe cases the tracheal and bronchial mucosa may also become involved. Minimal trauma during excision is required because of the recurrent nature of the lesions and the need for repeated removal.

Conservative treatment can be used if papillomas are small and non-symptomatic.

Cold steel excision may lead to scarring.

Microdebrider removal minimises scarring of the underlying tissue.

CO_2 laser removal has high thermal energy, which could cause more scarring.

Injection of lesions with anti-viral agents such as cidofovir has previously been used but may have carcinogenic effects. Medical therapy with interferon has also been used but it has a high risk of side effects.

Tracheostomy may be used for severe cases but it is associated with pulmonary seeding and has potential tracheotomy complications.

iv.   Cervical cancer prevention schemes use HPV immunisation with Gardasil (HPV 6, 11, 16, 18). Immunisation with Cervarix (HPV 16, 18) will not cover the HPV types implicated in recurrent respiratory papillomatosis. These will not help the current generation but may prevent vertical transmission of HPV during child birth.

CASE 31

A 38-year-old teacher presented with a 6-week history of hoarse voice. He also has a history of reflux disease. Endoscopic examination is shown in the picture.

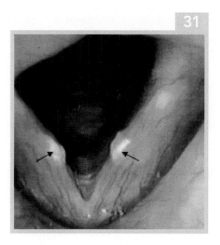

i.   What is this condition?

ii.   What is the initial best treatment?

iii. What is the best treatment if the condition persists?

iv.   What are GRBAS and VHI?

i.   Bilateral nodules affecting the anterior third of both true vocal folds.

ii.   This condition is common in professional voice users such as teachers, singers and public speakers as well as in children. Voice therapy including voice hygiene and anti-reflux treatment is usually sufficient to relieve this condition but needs cooperation from the patients.

iii.   If the nodules persist, surgical excision should be considered only after a thorough non-surgical treatment regimen is unsuccessful. Complications of surgical intervention, including permanent change in voice quality should be clearly explained to the patient.

iv.   GRBAS is an auditory-perceptual evaluation method for hoarseness. It is a subjective assessment of the degree and quality of hoarseness which scores (0–3) the grade of roughness, breathiness, asthenia and strain.

    VHI is the voice handicap index which patients use to subjectively evaluate social and lifestyle limitations (functional aspects), voice and larynx condition (physical aspects) and what the patient is feeling (emotional aspects).

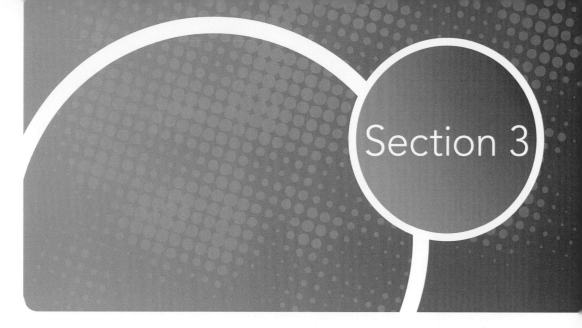

Section 3

OTOLOGY AND SKULL BASE

CASE 32

QUESTIONS 32

A 75-year-old gentleman attends out patients 7 days following a procedure.

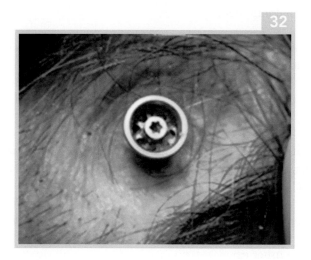

i.   What does the image show?

ii.   What are the indications?

iii. What are the common complications?

Answers 32

i. This photograph shows the abutment of a bone anchored hearing aid (BAHA) produced by Cochlear. This is one type of bone anchored hearing device (BAHD) although there are a number of other similar products on the market.

BAHDs have 3 components:

1. A titanium screw that, when placed in the skull, becomes firmly osseointegrated.

2. Either a percutaneous abutment or a subcutaneous metal plate that attach to the screw.

3. A vibrating external hearing aid. For the percutaneous implant, this hearing aid clips on to the abutment. For the intact skin implant, the hearing aid attaches using a strong magnet.

Sound is detected by the external hearing aid and converted to vibrations. These vibrations are transferred to the abutment or metal plate. They then pass through the skull to the inner ear.

ii. There are two main indications for BAHDs.

1. Conductive or mixed hearing loss in patients that are unable to use traditional hearing aids. The BAHD bypasses the conductive mechanism of the affected ear by transferring vibrations directly to the cochlea and is an excellent means of augmenting conductive hearing loss. The more powerful forms of BAHD are also able to rehabilitate mixed hearing losses in which the sensorineural hearing loss component is up to 60 dBHL. For most patients, traditional hearing aids offer the same benefits but if the ear canal is absent or very narrow or if the use of traditional hearing aids causes otitis externa or mastoid infection (in those that have had mastoid surgery) then a BAHA is very helpful as it leaves the ear canal free.

2. Transfer of sound from the side of a dead ear to the functioning contralateral ear. In this role BAHDs act in a similar way to a CROS aid. It allows individuals with a dead ear to hear sounds more effectively on the ipsilateral side through transcranial transmission to the contralateral ear. Whilst this is helpful to some extent, it does not actually restore hearing in the affected ear and therefore does not restore directional hearing or improve the ability to hear in a noisy environment, 2 situations in which those with unilateral hearing loss struggle.

iii. For the percutaneous type of BAHD, the most common complication is a soft-tissue reaction around the abutment (skin hypertrophy or complete overgrowth over the abutment), which can lead to problems attaching the external sound processor. Treatment includes topical steroid cream/injections, revision surgery to remove the excess skin or use of a longer length of abutment. This type of problem has become less frequent in recent years as local skin thinning and depilation around the abutment is no longer performed. The intact skin implants do not have this complication but can cause local skin necrosis because of prolonged pressure effects from the magnet. Failure of osseointegration is also an infrequent complication resulting in extrusion of the titanium screw. Complications are more common in children who are more likely to sustain trauma to the implant.

CASE 33

A 5-year-old child presents with a swollen right eye that has developed over 48 hours following an upper respiratory tract infection.

A computed tomography (CT) scan is requested.

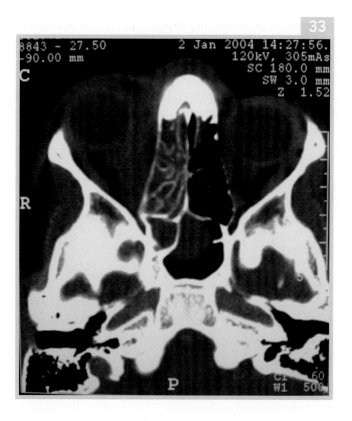

i.   What does the scan show?

ii.   How would you manage this child?

iii. What surgical approach would you use?

i. This axial CT scan demonstrates a right-sided subperiosteal abscess and opacification of right ethmoidal cells. There is also some proptosis of the right eye. This is a class III orbital cellulitis according to Chandler's classification.

ii. This child needs to be managed in a multidisciplinary setting. The paediatric and ophthalmology teams should be involved in the child's care. It is important to try and assess eye function. In older children visual acuity using a Snellen chart and colour vision using Ishihara charts can be assessed. Loss of colour vision is the first sign of impending ocular damage. In younger children this is not possible but a measure of ocular function can be made by assessing for an afferent pupillary defect. Light shone in the affected eye results in less pupillary constriction than light shone in the normal eye. Ocular movements should also be assessed if possible. It is also important to ensure that there is no intracranial complications from the infection. This may present with headache, meningism or reduced conscious level. The scan may identify a significant intracranial collection.

The child should be prescribed nasal decongestants and started on intravenous antibiotics according to local protocols as well as intravenous fluids. The definitive treatment for subperiosteal abscess is, however, surgical drainage.

iii. There are two options:

Open approach via Lynch–Howarth incision
An incision is performed on the medial orbital rim down to bone being wary of the angular vein. The orbital periosteum is elevated down to the pus collection and the pus gently evacuated. A drain is then inserted that is removed once drainage is minimal.

Endoscopic decompression
The abscess can be drained endonasally. This may, however, be more challenging in the presence of acute infection and inflammation. A combined external and endonasal procedure can also be performed.

CASE 34

A 15-year-old boy presents with a fluctuant swelling in front of his left ear. There is a visible pit.

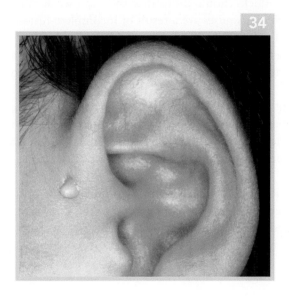

i.   What is the diagnosis?

ii.   What is the embryological origin of this condition?

iii. What is the treatment?

iv.   Define the terms cyst, sinus and fistula.

Answers 34

i.   Pre–auricular abscess.

ii. The first and second branchial arches each give rise to three hillocks adjacent to the dorsal end of the first branchial cleft; these structures are called the hillocks of His. These hillocks should unite after the sixth week of gestation to form the pinna. Pre–auricular sinuses are a result of incomplete fusion of these hillocks. They consist of a sinus opening on the preauricular skin and a subcutaneous network of tracts extending from the opening into adjacent tissues. In most cases these do not cause any problems but they may result in cyst or abscess formation.

iii. Any significant abscess requires surgical drainage and either oral or intravenous antibiotics depending on the severity of the infection. Once the infection is settled a wide local excision of the sinus opening and its subcutaneous tracts back to normal tissue is required to avoid recurrence.

iv. A cyst is an epithelium lined structure with no external opening. A sinus is an epithelium lined structure with an opening to the skin or to the gut. A fistula is an epithelialised connection from two epithelialised surfaces (indicating that the branchial cleft remnant has communicated to its corresponding branchial pouch remnant).

CASE 35

QUESTIONS 35

A 55-year-old woman presents with clear otorrhoea from her right ear. She has had multiple mastoid surgeries in the past for cholesteatoma, the last one about 20 years ago. She has intermittent clear otorrhea from her right ear several times a year since then. On examination, she has a large right mastoid cavity, with a skin-lined mass in the posterior superior aspect, easily seen through the wide meatoplasty (see picture).

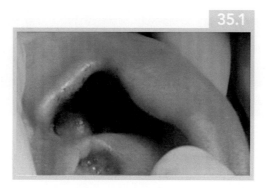

A magnetic resonance imaging (MRI) scan is performed, and representative coronal T1 and T2 images are shown below.

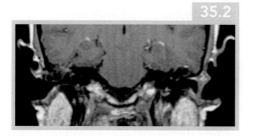

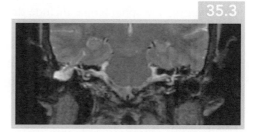

i.   What is the likely diagnosis? What clinical features on examination would make you suspicious of this diagnosis?

ii.   What are the most common causes of this disorder?

iii.   What are the surgical treatment options for this disorder?

Answers 35

i. The likely diagnosis is a meningoencephalocoele (brain hernia) into the right mastoid cavity. In this case, the T2 images suggest that the contents of the hernia are primarily cerebrospinal fluid (CSF). In other cases, the hernia is primarily full of brain tissue which is devitalised and non-functional. An example of a meningoencephalocoele containing more brain tissue is shown below (left hand side).

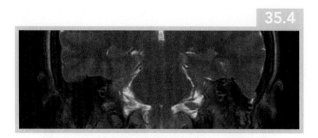

35.4

The clues on physical exam are that the mass arises superiorly, may expand on Valsalava and may be pulsatile. There may be associated CSF serous otitis media. The presence of CSF can be confirmed by testing the otorrohoea for tau-protein.

ii. Meningoencephalocoles can be congenital or acquired, with the latter being far more common. The most common etiology is previous mastoid surgery with damage to both the bony tegmen and the dura. Other causes of acquired meningoencephalocoele include destructive middle ear disease such as cholesteatoma, temporal bone fracture and benign intracranial hypertension. The latter occurs in overweight females in their third and fourth decades. Congenital meningoencephalocoeles may occur as a result of incomplete fusion of the skull bones during development or because of the presence of aberrant arachnoid granulations.

iii. Surgical options include transmastoid repair, middle fossa repair or combined middle fossa and transmastoid repair. Defects smaller than 15mm situated posterior to the ossicular chain are ideal for a transmastoid approach. A middle fossa approach is used for large or multiple defects and for defects that overlying the ossicular heads. The meningoencephalocoele can be amputated flush with the bony defect as the herniated brain tissue is non-functional. A triple layer repair is usually undertaken with a lining for the dura (eg. fascia or artificial dural replacement), a relatively rigid replacement for tegmen (eg. autologous cartilage, bone or a bone dust and fibrin glue patty) and a further layer of reinforcement to the mastoid surface (eg. temporalis fascia). Occasionally obliteration of the Eustachian tube oriface with or without blind sac closure can be used as an alternative technique, particularly if the ear has no hearing.

CASE 36

QUESTIONS 36

A 63-year-old man has a left-sided percutaneous bone-anchored hearing aid (BAHA) placed for conductive hearing loss. Five months later, he returns because he is unable to use the BAHA processor anymore. On inspection of the site, the following photograph illustrates what is seen.

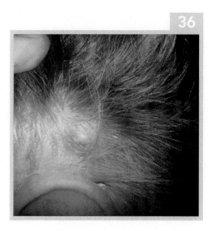

i.   What has occurred in this patient?

ii.   How are skin reactions around osseointegrated percutaneous classified and graded?

iii. What treatment options are available to prevent recurrence of such a complication if this is treated?

i. The skin has overgrown the abutment of the implanted device and completely covered it.

ii. Skin reactions around such osseointegrated bone conduction devices are typically graded according to Holger's classification. The gradings are as follows:

Grade 0: no reaction of skin

Grade 1: redness with slight swelling of skin around the abutment

Grade 2: redness, moistness and moderate swelling of skin around the abutment

Grade 3: presence of granulation tissue in addition to redness, moistness and moderate swelling with around the abutment

Grade 4: overt infection resulting in removal of the implant

iii. Options to consider when revising include: (1) using a longer abutment, (2) thinning skin and removing hair follicles and (3) intraoperative use of steroid injections. Post-operatively, topical steroid creams and steroid injections can also be considered in addition to pressure dressings and good local hygiene.

CASE 37

A 25-year-old man presents with a one-year history of a draining right ear with greenish discharge with odour. He has been complaining in the last week of increasing headaches and of fevers. On examination, the patient was noted to have a temperature of 38.8°C, an inflamed eardrum with greenish discharge through a perforation and some photophobia, but without meningeal signs. A computed tomography (CT) of the mastoid and brain with contrast was performed along with a magnetic resonance imaging (MRI) of the brain.

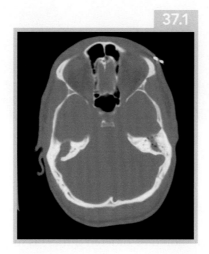

37.1

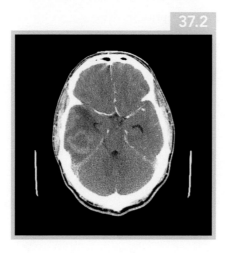

37.2

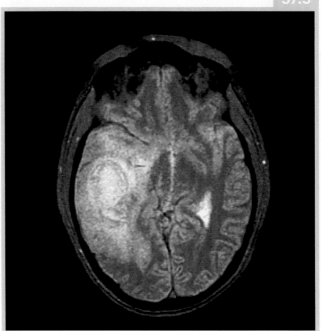

i. What is the diagnosis and what are the most common intracranial locations for this kind of lesion?

ii. At which point should lumbar puncture be performed, if at all?

iii. What kind of CT scan should be ordered if there is suspicion of brain abscess?

iv. What are the management options?

Answers 37

i. The diagnosis is otogenic brain abscess. The opacified mastoid antrum can be seen in the first CT scan. The second brain window scan shows a rim-enhancing lesion in the temporal bone, confirmed by the MRI, which also shows the surrounding oedema. The most common site of an otogenic abscess is the temporal lobe followed by the cerebellum. Subdural empyema may also form but is less common.

ii. If there is suspicion of possible increased intracranial pressure, a lumbar puncture should not be performed until this is ruled out with a CT scan. Lumbar puncture in this situation can lead to 'coning' as the brain prolapses inferiorly under pressure.

iii. If a brain abscess is suspected, bone window CT scan is not sufficient, brain soft-tissue windows should be used and contrast should be requested, as an abscess may be missed without contrast. The ventricles should also be examined for dilation, an indicator of increased intracranial pressure.

iv. There is no universally accepted treatment algorithm. If there is progressive deterioration due to increased intracranial pressure, the brain abscess should be drained either via craniotomy or CT-guided aspiration. Many authors recommend trial of intravenous antibiotics first with careful monitoring of the abscess radiologically and clinically. The timing of the mastoid surgery can follow treatment of the abscess or can be concurrent if there is surgical management of the abscess planned.

CASE 38

QUESTIONS 38

A 47-year-old man presents with headaches, mild ataxia and numbness of the right side of his face. He has a positive head thrust test (head impulse test) to the right side.

He has a electronystagmogram (ENG) performed to investigate this further, which shows the responses illustrated. The next figure shows his horizontal eye lead recordings on gaze directed to the right side and to the left side.

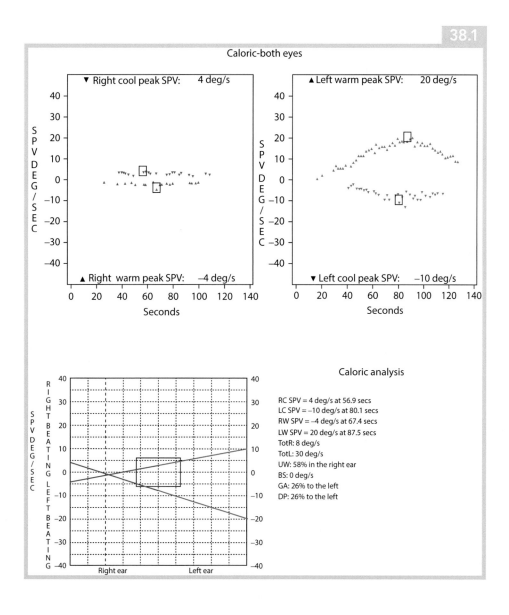

38.1

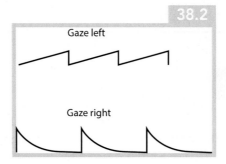

i.   What does the caloric testing show? What is the formula for calculating caloric asymmetry?

ii.   Describe the type of nystagmus shown, its name and its underlying pathophysiology.

iii. What other neurological findings may be seen with this?

Answers 38

i. Shown is a typical caloric report. The top graph shows slow-phase velocities (SPVs) to warm and cold irrigation (blue left ear, red right ear) showing the typical low frequency response to warm and cold (30°C and 42°C) irrigations over the time course of the irrigation. The lower plot shows a 'butterfly' plot, showing peak SPV in both ears to warm and cold irrigation. A significant asymmetry in responses is shown with the right ear being hypo-responsive. The formula for calculating asymmetry is the Jongkee's formula:

$$\frac{\left(\left(\text{Right Warm SPV} + \text{Right Cold SPV}\right) - \left(\text{Left Warm SPV} + \text{Left Cold SPV}\right)\right)}{\left(\text{Right Warm SPV} + \text{Right Cold SPV} + \text{Left Warm SPV} + \text{Left Cold SPV}\right)}$$

ii. The gaze tracings show a saw-tooth type left beating nystagmus to left gaze with linear slow ramps to the slow phases. The nystagmus is direction changing and shows a right beating nystagmus to right gaze with non-linear saddle-shaped slow phases. This is typical of Brun's nystagmus, which is generated in the presence of a large cerebellopontine angle (CPA) lesion.

The saw-tooth left beating nystagmus arises from the vestibular loss on the right side and is more marked on looking to the left because of Alexander's Law and because central static compensation mechanisms are disrupted by brainstem and cerebellar compression. The right beating non-linear ramp nystagmus is typical gaze-evoked nystagmus and is caused by loss of the neural integrator which maintains eccentric gaze position after saccades to eccentric eye positions. This occurs because of the cerebellar and brainstem compression on the right side.

Lesions, such as the one below, a very large vestibular schwannoma, can cause this type of nystagmus

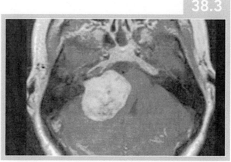

38.3

iii. Other neurological findings that may be seen are impaired or saccadic smooth pursuit, cerebellar signs such as intention tremor or ataxia, facial nerve weakness and trigeminal sensory loss (seen in this case). Large tumours may also cause hydrocephalus with all its attendant neurological manifestations.

CASE 39

QUESTIONS 39

A 78-year-old woman presents to the emergency department complaining of a severe sense of spinning, vomiting and ataxia. She can barely sit up in the stretcher but is oriented and answers questions appropriately. This has been going on continuously for about 4 hours and this is the first time she has had this kind of episode. She has an occipital headache and no subjective hearing loss confirmed by tuning fork tests. Past history includes a history of hypertension and previous myocardial infarction.

She has nystagmus which is left beating on left gaze and right beating on right gaze. Her head thrust testing is negative to both sides. Her smooth pursuit tracing is shown as follows.

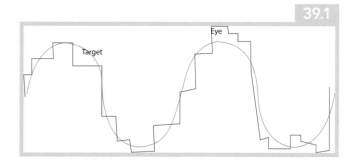

A computed tomography (CT) and magnetic resonance imaging (MRI) scan has been performed.

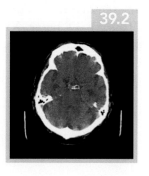

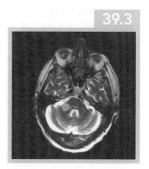

i.   What does the smooth pursuit tracing show?

ii.   What is the likely diagnosis and what do these scans show?

iii. What other clinical tests can help to distinguish this condition from an inner ear condition?

i.   The tracing shows severely saccadic smooth pursuit. This is a non-localising
      finding, generally associated with central nervous system (CNS) pathology,
      although it can occur with some drugs, such as anticonvulsants. Milder saccadic
      smooth pursuit is normal with ageing.

ii.   This patient likely has central vertigo from a brainstem/cerebellar lesion. She has
      several vascular risk factors (age, hypertension, previous myocardial infarction
      [MI]). Her CT and MRI scans show an ischemic stroke in the right brainstem/
      cerebellar peduncle. She demonstrates direction-changing nystagmus.

iii. There are several features that would point to a brainstem/cerebellar aetiology.
      The head thrust test is particularly useful. In this test, the head is moved with
      high velocity to one direction and, if the vestibule-ocular reflex on that side
      is impaired, there will be a corrective saccade back to the target at the end of
      the head movement. The acronym HINS is a useful aid memoire. This stands
      for head impulse, no skew. Vertigo and nystagmus from a peripheral aetiology
      should be associated with a positive head impulse test to the affected side, and,
      if this is not present, this is worrisome. Skew deviation is found when one eye is
      positioned lower than the other and covering and uncovering both eyes reveals
      that one eye has to elevate to acquire the target. Other findings to look for are
      cerebellar signs (dysdiadokinesia, past pointing, intention tremor), a Horner
      syndrome (pupillary miosis, partial ptosis, ahydrosis and enophthalmos), signs
      of spinothalamic tract involvement (crossed facial and body loss to pinprick,
      loss of temperature sensation in contralateral body) and loss of facial sensation
      on ipsilateral side through involvement of the sensory nucleus of the Vth nerve.
      The spino-cererebellar, sensory V nerve, VII nerve, IX nerve, XI nerve,
      spinothalamic and sympathetic tracts are all in the lateral brainstem.

QUESTIONS 40

A 42-year-old woman presents with a history of progressive hearing loss. Her audiogram is shown. As shown on the audiogram, she has no contralateral reflexes on the left side to the sound presentation on the right side and a questionable reflex at 110 dB HL at 2 kHz on the right ipsilateral testing. On left-sided sound presentation, she has good ipsilateral reflexes and reflexes are also present in the right ear and the traces are shown (up is a decrease in admittance in these tracings).

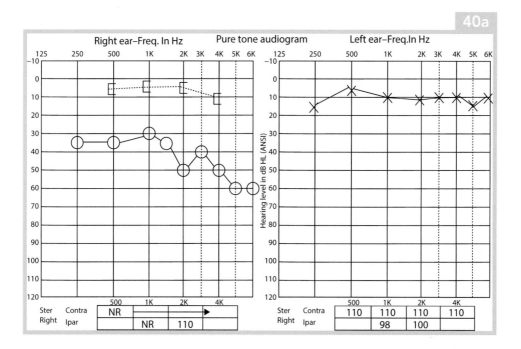

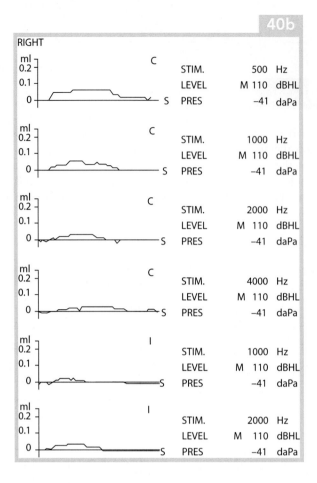

i.   What is unusual in this audiogram?

ii. What conditions may result in this kind of pattern?

i. The unusual finding is that reflexes, although somewhat elevated, are clearly present in the right ear on left-sided sound stimulation, as seen in the reflex tracings at most frequencies. This is very unusual with this level of conductive hearing loss and is not in keeping with otosclerosis. It implies that the effector arm (the stapedius) is still able to manifest its action, that is, the process causing the conductive hearing loss has not changed the mobility of the ossicular chain. Appropriately, because of the conductive hearing loss on the right side, there are no contralateral reflexes.

ii. Several conditions can cause a conductive hearing loss with preserved stapedial reflexes. The simplest cause is a calibration error in the bone or air conduction transducers. In this situation, the stimulation level of the bone or air conduction transducer is not accurately reported on the audiometer reading, and it can artefactually appear that the air and bone conductions thresholds are different, when in fact they are not. Calibration errors typically manifest as a milda mild conductive hearing loss, and miscalibration seen to the extent shown here would be very unusual. Other causes are fracture or loss of the stapes suprastructure medial to the insertion of the stapedius tendon. In this case, stapedius contraction is able to cause stiffening of the incus/malleus/eardrum but the loss of suprastructure results in failure of transmission of this stiffening to the stapes footplate. A more common cause to consider in clinical practice is superior canal dehiscence (SCD). This can cause a conductive hearing loss which can be marked and can resemble the audiogram in otosclerosis. Most often, however, SCD cause a "pseudoconductive" hearing loss only in the low frequencies on audiometry, partly caused by better than normal bone conduction hearing thresholds (e.g. thresholds at −10dB HL), and slightly reduced air conduction hearing thresholds. Other inner ear abnormalities such as x-linked stapes gusher syndrome and enlarged vestibular aqueduct can cause a non-middle ear related hearing loss. In these cases it is thought that the pressure in the vestibule exerted on the stapes footplate acts to stiffen it and increase its mechanical input impedance, similar to stiffening of the annular ligament in otosclerosis. Non-organic hearing loss, in which a subject is falsifying their true hearing thresholds can also cause a mismatch in the air and bone conduction hearing thresholds manifesting as an air-bone gap. Sometimes this can even be a reversed air-bone gap, with air conduction better than bone conduction.

In this particular case, it was caused by necrosis of the stapes arch below the stapes head, probably from this patient's multiple childhood infections. This caused some attenuation of the mechanical transmission to the stapes footplate and the conductive loss seen, but because the stapes head was still intact and connected to the tympanic membrane by the incus and malleus, stapedial contraction still results in stiffening of the eardrum and an intact stapedial reflex.

CASE 41

QUESTIONS 41

A 46-year-old man presents with a sensation of pressure in his left ear and two episodes of otorrohoea from his left ear. His ear exam is normal, as is his audiogram. A computed tomography (CT) scan of the temporal bones is taken and, based on this, MRI scans are performed.

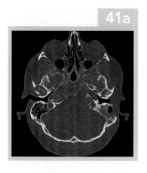
41a

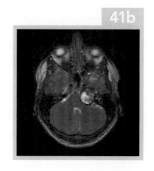
41b

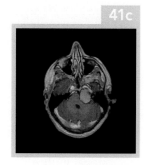
41c

i. What imaging MRI sequences are used in scans 2 and 3?

ii. What is the differential diagnosis for the appearance of the CT scan in 39a?

iii. What is the likely diagnosis after reviewing the MRI images in 39b and c?

iv. What surgical management approaches are clinically used to manage this lesion?

i. T2-weighted sequence is shown in 39b as fluid in the globe of the eye and cerebrospinal fluid (CSF) are hyperintense. T1-weighted sequence with gadolinium enhancement is shown in 39c. CSF is dark, subcutaneous fat is bright, retro-orbital fat (not seen in this image) would also be bright and the turbinates and mucosal lining of the nose is bright.

ii. This shows a destructive process in the petrous apex, relatively smooth walled and expansile looking. Other differential diagnoses in the petrous apex include epidermoid or congenital cholesteatoma, chondrosarcoma, chordoma (although these are usually midline, they can expand laterally), mucocoele and petrous apicitis.

iii. This lesion appears to be hyperintense on T1- and T2-weighted images, even without contrast on T1. The most likely diagnosis is that of cholesterol granuloma, proven in this case at surgery. It is not uncommon to have variable signal within the cyst rather than a homogenous appearing cyst. The signal characteristics on MRI of a cholesterol granuloma are often the same as retained petrous apex secretions but cholesterol granulomas produce expansion and breakdown of bony trabeulae whereas retained secretions do not.

iv. Surgical approaches to CG can be divided into those that do not preserve hearing and those that do. Many approaches are designed to only drain the cyst. The hearing destructive approaches may be valid if hearing is already loss and include translabyrinthine and transcochlear approaches. Hearing preservation approaches can be divided into transpetrous, middle fossa and trans-sphenoid. The transpetrous approaches include the infracochlear approach (below the cochlea between the carotid and jugular bulb), the infralabyrinthine (below the posterior semicircular canal, deep to the facial nerve and superior to the jugular bulb) and the partial labyrinthectomy approaches (usually through the superior canal with plugging of the remaining labyrinth). Occasionally, other approaches such as the transcrural approach (through the arch of the superior semicircular canal) or anterior subtemporal approaches have been described. The middle fossa approach is self-evident and is much more effective at removing the lining of the cyst in recurrent cases. Trans-sphenoid approaches are gaining popularity, even in those cases in which the sphenoid does not abut the cyst; some of the skull base can be drilled endoscopically to reach the cyst.

A 40-year-old woman complains of increasing hearing loss for over 15 years. Her audiogram is shown as follows.

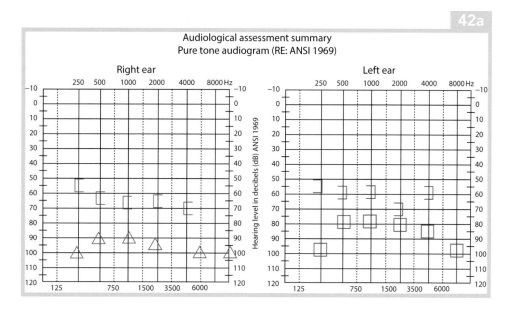

She also undergoes computed tomography (CT) scanning of the temporal bones. The scans are shown as follows.

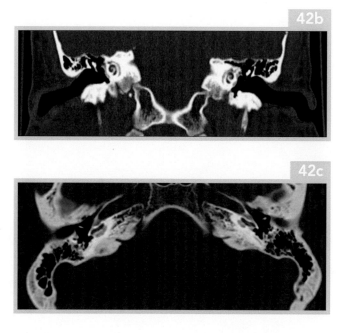

i.   What is the likely diagnosis?

ii.   What treatment options are available for hearing stabilisation?

iii. What are the treatment options for hearing rehabilitation?

iv.   The patient eventually undergoes cochlear implantation. What are the special risks of cochlear implantation in this condition?

i.   The diagnosis is otosclerosis with cochlear involvement or fenestral and cochlear otosclerosis. The 'double ring' sign around the cochlea on CT is typical of this disease. Osteogenesis imperfecta can lead to a similar CT appearance but is far less common in the temporal bone.

ii. Various drug treatment strategies have been proposed for stabilising hearing with inner-ear involvement. There are several studies (although relatively low grade) suggesting that fluoride treatment may slow the progression of sensorineural hearing loss, although the dosage and treatment duration is very heterogenous in these studies. More recently, bisphosphonates, particularly third-generation bisphosphonates, such as zoledronate or risedronate, have been suggested to be useful in stabilising hearing as well.

iii. Hearing rehabilitation options always include standard hearing aids. In this case, consideration should strongly be given to stapedotomy to close the air-bone gap followed by hearing aids. This would allow much better function with the hearing aids. The third option is cochlear implantation. At this level of hearing, this might well be considered if hearing is not satisfactory with hearing aids even after stapedotomy or stapedectomy. Another possible option is to drive the inner ear with a middle ear driver such as the CODACS™ driver from Cochlear Corp, which bypasses the footplate with a stapedotomy.

iv. There are special challenges in cochlear implantation of ears such as this. Implantation has been reported into the false otosclerotic demineralised lumen, which surrounds the cochlea as the 'double ring'. The round window may be obliterated by otosclerosis, making finding landmarks difficult. Intracochlear fibrosis or ossification of the basal turn may require drilling out this segment. After implantation, there is a higher risk of facial nerve cross stimulation in this disorder, particularly for the distal electrodes.

CASE 43

A 19-year-old woman presents complaining of a several year history of hearing a chronic noise in her right ear, which she has been hearing for several years in time with her heartbeat. It is present all the time but worse in quiet. She does not complain of any hearing loss or vertigo. The following image is what you see when you look in her ear. The computed tomography (CT) scan and magnetic resonance angiogram (MRA) are also shown.

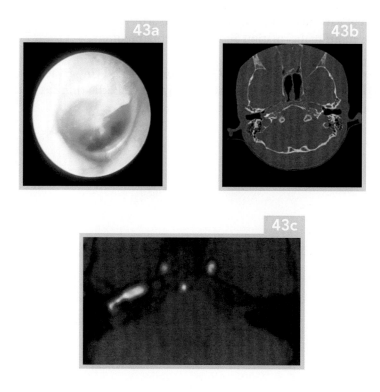

i.   What is the likely diagnosis?

ii.   What is the differential diagnosis from the ear examination alone?

iii. How should this be managed?

i.   This shows an ectopic and dehiscent carotid artery. Although in the CT scan it appears the carotid and jugular bulb are connected, this is not actually the case.

ii.   The differential diagnosis from the clinical appearance alone would include glomus tympanicum or jugulare, vascular middle ear tumour such as middle ear adenoma and dehiscent jugular bulb, although that would not be quite as bright red. A glomus tumour might blanche on applying pressure to the external ear canal (Brown's sign). Other less common lesions that could be mistaken for a dehiscent carotid are a persistent stapedial artery, carotid artery aneurysm, arterio-venous malformation and cholesterol granuloma.

iii. In almost all cases, this condition should be managed conservatively. Occasionally patients are very distressed by the pulsatile tinnitus but this cannot easily be resolved with any surgical management.

CASE 44

A 39-year-old man presents with twitching of the left side of his face and subjective hearing loss on the left. On examination, he has mild synkinesis of the left side of his face and myokymia with slightly delayed blink on the left side. His ear exam shows a hint of a reddish mass in the middle through the eardrum. His audiogram is shown as follows.

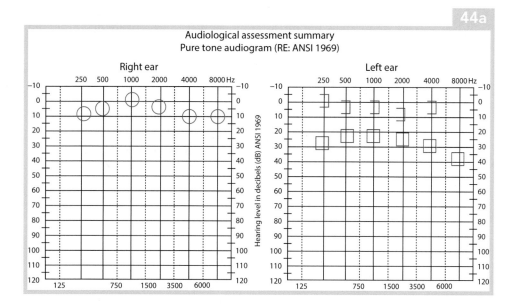

He undergoes computed tomography (CT) scanning and magnetic resonance imaging (MRI) scanning. Scans are shown as follows.

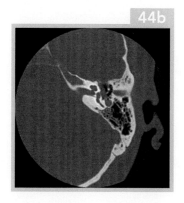

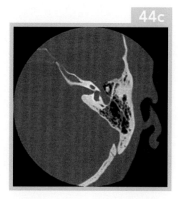

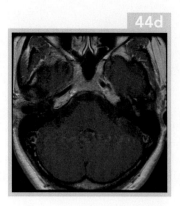

44d

i.   What does the audiogram and imaging show? What is the likely diagnosis and how would you confirm it in this man?

ii. Where does this lesion most often occur?

iii. What is the differential diagnosis in this radiologic lesion?

iv. What is the best management option for this man currently and, if the facial function starts to deteriorate, in the future?

i.   The audiogram shows a mild conductive hearing loss in the left ear. The CT scans show considerable expansion of the horizontal and upper vertical portions of the facial nerve. There does not appear to be significant expansion of the geniculate ganglion, labyrinthine portion of the facial nerve or of the internal auditory canal. It is not possible to say whether the nerve is abnormal more distally as there are no more inferior slices available. On the T1 weighted MRI image with gadolinium there is enhancement of the expanded nerve and this appears to extend to the greater superficial petrosal nerve.

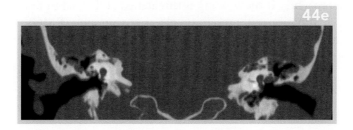

44e

The likely diagnosis with this presentation and imaging is a schwannoma of the mastoid portion of the facial nerve. The diagnosis is based on the clinical and radiological findings and this lesion should NOT be biopsied, unless malignancy is suspected for other reasons (e.g. malignant parotid mass).

ii.   Facial nerve schwannomas most often occur at the geniculate ganglion. A more typical imaging appearance is shown below on a gadolinium-enhanced T1-weighted MRI image. This shows a lesion involving the right geniculate ganglion and the internal auditory canal.

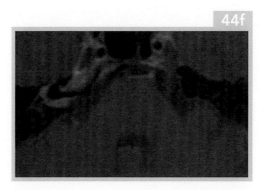

44f

iii.   The most common lesion of the facial nerve in the middle ear and mastoid segment is a schwannoma. Haemangiomas can also occur but usually occur around the geniculate ganglion. They can cause bony spiculation on the CT scan and are then called ossifying haemangiomas. Other lesions can spread from the parotid to the mastoid facial nerve, such as adenoid cystic tumours, or squamous tumours of the parotid or external ear canal. Paragangliomas along the facial canal have been rarely described as well.

iv.   There is minimal facial nerve weakness currently. The synkinesis shows, however, that there is a process of degeneration and regeneration that has been present for some time. The best management at this stage is conservative with observation. If the facial nerve function begins to deteriorate, there are various options but no definitively accepted solution. These options include stereotactic radiosurgery to prevent further growth of the schwannoma, decompression of the facial nerve schwannoma, partial debulking of the lesion and combinations of these approaches. If the hearing is threatened and facial function is poor, but facial muscle function still present on electromyography (EMG) testing, then resection and restoration of nerve continuity by a nerve graft or hypoglossal/facial crossover cable graft are other options.

CASE 45

QUESTIONS 45

A 55-year-old man complains of increasing bilateral hearing loss. His audiogram is shown as follows. The patient undergoes a computed tomography (CT) scan of the temporal bones. Two cuts are shown.

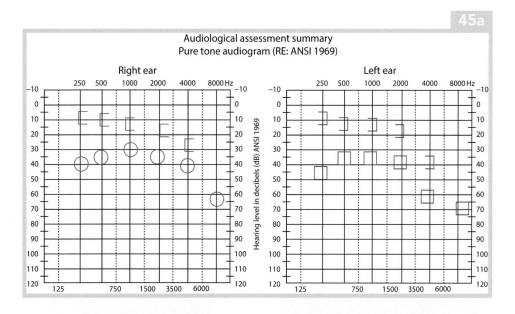

45a

Audiological assessment summary
Pure tone audiogram (RE: ANSI 1969)

Right ear / Left ear

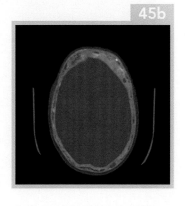

45b

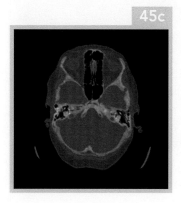

45c

i.   What is the likely diagnosis and how could this be confirmed?

ii.   What is the differential diagnosis of radiologically diffuse involvement of the temporal bone?

i. With the mixed hearing loss seen on the audiogram and the diffuse bilateral involvement of the calvarium seen on the CT scan, the most likely diagnosis is Paget's disease. This diagnosis can be strongly suspected from the CT appearance, with the washed out and fluffy appearance of the bone and with an apparent increase in calvarial bone volume. The CT scan may also show osteoporosis circumscripta, which are round, punched-out lesions, seen primarily in the frontal bones and occur in 10%–15% of patients. Other helpful tests are Technetium[99] bone scans, which may show widespread skeletal involvement, and the biochemical markers alkaline phosphatase and urinary hydroxyproline, which are often elevated. Serum calcium is normal. Acid phosphatase may be elevated in about 20% of patients.

ii. Diffuse involvement of the temporal bone can occur in various diseases including fibrous dysplasia, osteogenesis imperfecta, otosclerosis, osteopetrosis, osteoblastic metastatic lesions from the prostate, otosyphilis and Camurati–Engelmann disease (progressive diaphyseal dysplasia). Rarely do these disorders actually result in an increase in apparent volume of bone but rather demineralisation and remodelling of bone. Fibrous dysplasia can show a typical 'ground glass' CT appearance. CT scans shown are of fibrous dysplasia and osteogenesis imperfecta of the temporal bone.

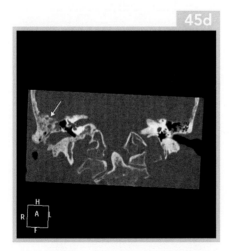

45d

Right temporal bone fibrous dysplasia

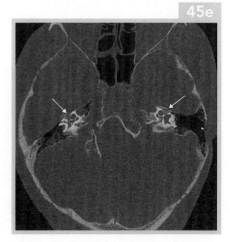

45e

Bilateral osteogenesis imperfecta affecting the temporal bones

CASE 46

QUESTIONS 46

A 30-year-old woman presents with a left-sided pulsatile tinnitus, dizziness on straining and autophony. Her audiogram is shown. 'R' represents stapedial reflex thresholds on the audiogram.

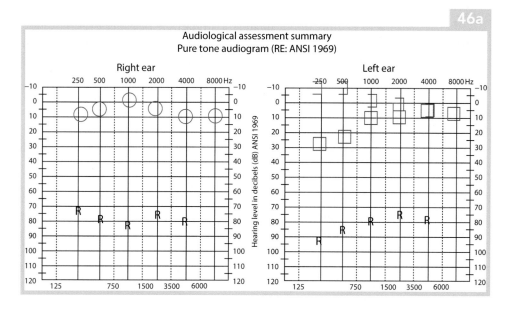

i. What is the likely diagnosis and what features on the audiogram would indicate this diagnosis?

ii. What other symptoms are typical of this disorder? What signs can be elicited on clinical examination to help confirm this diagnosis?

iii. What further tests could be performed to confirm the diagnosis?

i. The likely diagnosis is superior semicircular canal dehiscence (SCD). The features suggestive of this on the audiogram are: (1) mild conductive hearing loss in the low frequencies, (2) bone conduction thresholds less than zero (–10 dB, i.e. hypersensitive) in the low frequencies and (3) stapedial reflexes still present despite the conductive hearing loss.

ii. Other symptoms to enquire about include: (1) Does she hear her eyes moving when looking around in a quiet room? (2) Does she get dizzy with straining such as heavy lifting or when opening her bowels? (3) Does she get dizzy with loud environmental sounds (Tulio's phenomenon)? (4) Does she have a sensation of fullness in her ear? (5) Does she hear her footsteps resonating in her ear while walking or running?

All of these are typical symptoms of SCD. Non-specific lightheadedness can also occur.

On examination, findings may include: (1) the Weber's tuning fork test should strongly localise to the affected ear, (2) a low-frequency tuning fork (256 Hz or lower) placed on the ankle may be heard in the affected ear but not in the normal ear and (3) fistula testing may evoke a slow phase nystagmus that is directed upward and torsionally away from the pressurised ear with resetting downwards and torsion back to neutral eye position.

The figure shows the direction of the slow phase of eye movement on pressurisation of the left ear (s = superior, m = medial, l = lateral, i = inferior) indicated by the thick straight arrow.

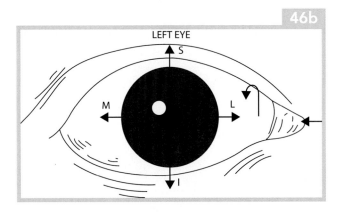

LEFT EYE

iii. Other tests that could be ordered include a fine-cut CT scan. This can be coronal, or reconstructed in the plane of the superior canal (Porschel's plane) or at 90° to the canal (Stenver's plane). The following image shows a coronal CT scan demonstrating bilateral SCD, which is also common (30%–40%).

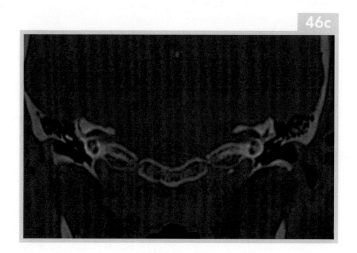

A second test commonly used to see if the SCD is functionally 'open' are the vestibular evoked myogenic potentials (VEMPs). These can be cervical or ocular but the cervical VEMPs are most commonly used. The following shows VEMP responses which are abnormally hypersensitive (present even at 65 dB nHL) in the left ear. The lowest level at which responses can be detected depends on the protocol used (tone bursts vs. clicks, frequency etc.), but both the right and left ears here show abnormally low thresholds.

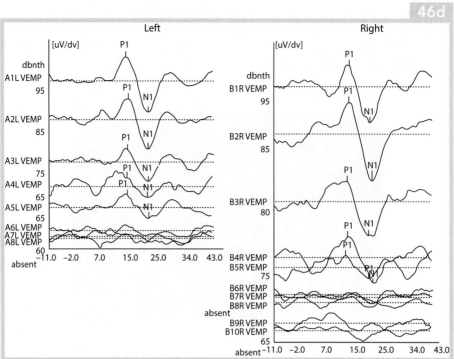

CASE 47

A 30-year-old woman presents with acute vertigo of sudden onset and present for 4 days. It is worse with head movements. She has been nauseated, vomiting and ataxic. There are no central neurological findings or symptoms but a nystagmus is seen in all eye positions. Audiogram and electronystagmogram (ENG) findings are shown as follows.

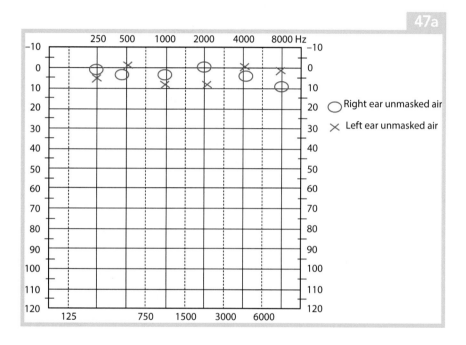

47a

Her ENG tracings below were recorded with the subject looking to the left (A), centre gaze (B) and to the right (C).

A: Left gaze – Horizontal leads

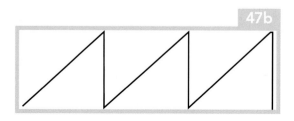

47b

B: Centre gaze – Horizontal leads

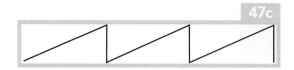

C: Right gaze – Horizontal leads

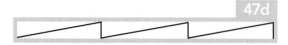

Vertical leads all gaze positions

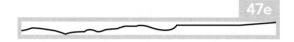

i.   What is the likely diagnosis?

ii.   What type of nystagmus do the ENG leads show? Which ear is the lesion in?

iii.   What law is illustrated in the ENG tracings?

i. The most likely diagnosis is vestibular neuronitis. There is nystagmus on the ENG and a normal audiogram. Vestibular neuronitis typically causes acute onset of vertigo, sometimes with a preceding upper respiratory tract infection, lasting for days at a time. The hearing is not affected, distinguishing it from sudden sensorineural hearing loss with vertigo (sometimes loosely called viral labyrinthitis); the vertigo is not episodic and is too long in duration for disorders, such as migraine-associated vertigo or Ménière's disease, which typically only last for hours. The following table classifies vertigo by hearing loss and duration. Another entity to consider, particularly in older adults, is a brainstem/cerebellar stroke. In that condition, other neurological signs, such as cranial nerve palsies, spinothalamic sensory signs, oculomotor findings, such as saccadic smooth pursuit and Horner syndrome may be seen.

Disorder	Duration of vertigo	Hearing loss	Positive head thrust sign
Vestibular neuronitis	Hours to days	No	Yes
Migraine-associated vertigo or recurrent vestibulopathy	Minutes to hours	No	No
Ménière's disease	Minutes to hours	Yes – may be fluctuant	Variable, no in early disease
BPPV	Seconds to minutes	No	No
SSNHL with vertigo	Hours to days	Yes	Yes – but can be variable
Brainstem stroke	Hours to days	No	No

ii. The ENG tracings show a purely horizontal nystagmus; typically there is a torsional component in acute peripheral loss but this can be difficult to capture on standard ENG. This is direction fixed and left beating. Since nystagmus beats towards the more active ear, and, in this case it is left beating, this implies a paresis of the right ear, so the lesion is in the right ear.

iii. The law illustrated is Alexander's law. This law implies that the nystagmus gets worse looking towards the fast phase of the nystagmus. It is generally associated with peripheral pathologies.

CASE 48

QUESTIONS 48

A 46-year-old man presents with right-sided tinnitus for several years. He has experienced mild unsteadiness as well. He finds he cannot use his phone in his right ear like he used to do in the past. His audiogram is shown below.

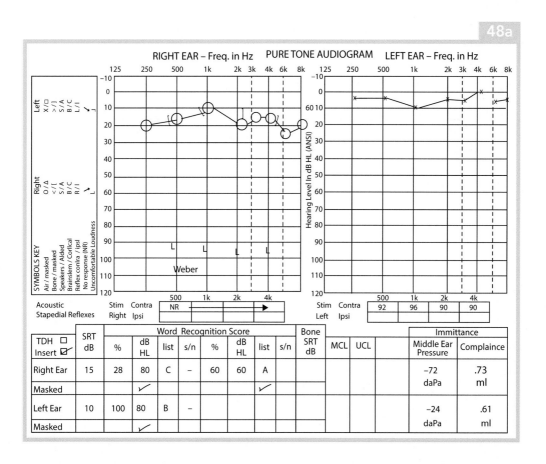

The word recognition score in the right ear is 28% and 100% in the left ear. Reflexes are shown as absent in the right ear. Distortion product OAEs are shown.

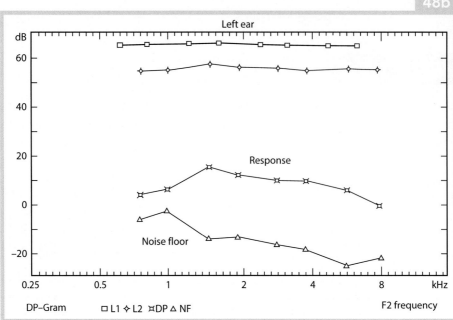

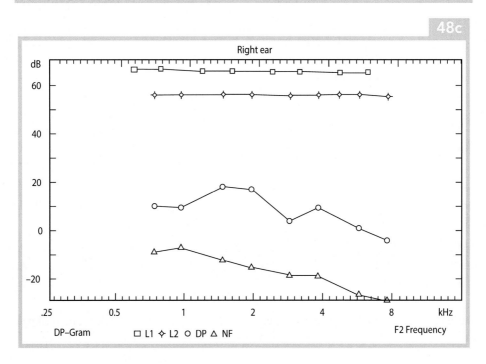

The patient underwent auditory brainstem evoked potential (ABR) testing shown as follows.

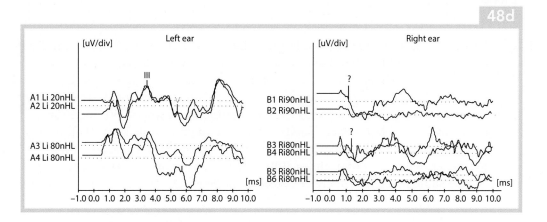

i.   What findings, if any, are suspicious in the audiogram for retrocochlear pathology? What other findings might there be in a standard audiogram (including reflex testing) to suggest retrocochlear pathology?

ii. What do the OAEs show and is this compatible with retrocochlear pathology?

iii. What does the ABR show and is this compatible with retrocochlear pathology?

iv. What are the limitations of the ABR in detecting vestibular schwannoma (VS)?

i. Despite the fact that the hearing is unusually well preserved in the right ear, the audiogram shows two findings suspicious for retrocochlear pathology: (1) a low word recognition score and (2) absent crossed reflexes on sound presentation to the right ear. Other findings that would be suspicious of retrocochlear pathology would be: (1) rollover, in which speech recognition gets worse with increasing presentation level of the speech and (2) reflex decay, the normal stapedial reflex to a 1 kHz stimulus decays in amplitude by less than 50% in 10 seconds (more for higher frequencies of stimulus). Other tests such as loudness balance tests or Bekesy audiometry are largely of historical interest now.

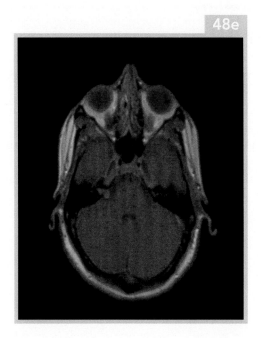

48e

This patient, in fact, did have a right VS, which is shown as follows.

ii. The OAE testing is normal. OAEs are normal in many patients with VS, more so if there is only mild hearing loss, but the exact percentage varies from study to study. In some studies up to 50% of subjects with VS have absent OAEs. This is suggestive that the VS may affect blood supply to the cochlea in about half of subjects. Present OAE does not rule in or rule out retrocochlear pathology.

iii. The ABR essentially shows absent waveforms in the right ear. The left ear waveforms look normal. This is consistent with a vestibular schwannoma.

iv.   There are several limitations to the ABR in the diagnosis of VS. First, if the hearing loss is marked (>70 dB at 4 kHz), there may be no responses at all even with purely cochlear hearing loss. Second, the sensitivity, while good overall at about 95% for all VS tumours, is lower for small tumours under 1 cm or intracanicular VS. While it may be around 85% overall for these tumours, in some studies it has been reported as having a sensitivity as low as 70% for these size tumours. With a specificity of around 80% and a low *a priori* probability that any given hearing loss is due to VS, this means that the positive predictive value of ABR is low for most hearing loss populations, as the vast majority will be false positives.

CASE 49

A 52-year-old woman presents with left sided hearing loss, tinnitus and occasional episodes of imbalance.

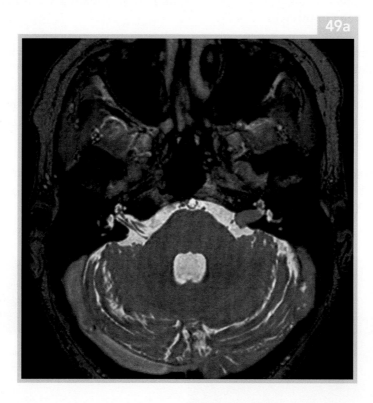

i.   What type of scan is shown and what is the primary abnormality?

ii.   What is the natural history of this abnormality?

iii. What is the differential diagnosis of this abnormality?

iv.   What are the treatment options for this abnormality and what are the pros and cons of each?

i. This scan is an axial T2-weighted MRI scan (FIESTA sequence) of the internal auditory meati showing a predominantly intracanlicular left sided vestibular schwannoma (VS). There is only a very small cerebellopontine angle (CPA) component. This type of scan is routinely used to monitor VS but, at some point, the patient should under go at least one T1-weighted MRI with gadolinium enhancement as this type of scan is helpful in differentiating VS from other types of pathology in this region.

ii. Only around 30% of VS demonstrate growth following diagnosis with a further 10% showing regression. Approximately 60% of VS remain stable. The reason why some tumours stop growing is unclear but it is likely that hormonal, cytokine or growth factor mediated mechanisms are responsible. Those tumours that grow tend to grow slowly with a mean annual increase in size of around 2 mm. They can, however, grow up to 15 mm per year.

iii. The table below summarises the differential diagnosis of a lesion within the CPA. It is divided into the different anatomical structures that are found within the CPA.

49b

Cisterns	Epidermoid cyst Dermoid cyst Lipoma Neurenteric cyst Neuroepithelial cyst	Meninges	Meningioma Arachnoid cyst Metastases
Arteries	Aneurysm Ectasia	Nerves	Cranial nerve schwannomas Malignant nerve sheath tumours
Skull base	Cholesterol granuloma Paraganglioma Chordoma Chondrosarcoma Endolymphatic sac tumour	Ventricles	Glioma Lymphoma Ependymoma Papilloma Haemangioblastoma Medulloblastoma

Vestibular schwannomas make up around 85% of CPA lesions. Approximately 5% are meningiomas. These have similar signal characteristics to VS but tend to be broad based, tend to be eccentric to the internal auditory canal and, with contrast enhancement, often demonstrate a dural tail. 2% are epidermoid tumours. These are congenital keratin cysts that slowly expand and surround the structures of the CPA. They are of high signal on T2-weighted MR imaging and low signal on T1-weighted imaging whether or not gadolinium is used. The diagnostic imaging modality is non-EPI MRI on which they have very high signal in comparison to all other forms of CPA pathology. Most types of pathology within the CPA have distinctive enough imaging characteristics to be able to make a radiological diagnosis. Malignant pathology is extremely rare with metastases making up by the far the largest pathology in this group.

iv. There are 3 main treatment modalities for sporadic VS.

1. Watch wait and rescan: This is a form of conservative management and is indicated in the vast majority of tumours as long as they are stable and smaller than 25 mm (maximum diameter in the CPA). This consists of serial imaging with the first scan 6 months following the diagnostic scan. This identifies any rapidly growing tumours. For the next 3 years scans should be undertaken annually. If there is no change in size then the interval between scans can be increased to every other year and eventually to every 3 years. If the tumour has been stable for 5 years then the chances of it ever growing become less than 5%. A conservative approach is the best way of preserving the patients medium term audiological function although it is likely that the hearing will gradually deteriorate over time (on average 2 dB per year).

2. Surgery: There are 3 main surgical approaches, namely the retrosigmoid (RS) approach, translabyrinthine (TL) approach and middle fossa approach. With the retrosigmoid approach any tumour, irrespective of size, can be removed. The approach is quick to perform and, if the tumour is small (<10 mm in the CPA) and there is CSF lateral to the tumour in the internal auditory canal, it may be possible to presrve hearing in those who have serviceable hearing at surgery. The TL approach also allows ny size tumour to be removed. It is not possible to preserve hearing with this approach as the vestibular apparatus is removed. It takes longer to perform than the RS approach but it allows good visualisation of the facial nerve both proximally and distally and does not require significant cerebellar retraction. The middle fossa approach only allows removal of tumours with a CPA component <10 mm. It is a hearing preservation approach but it has poorer facial nerve function outcomes than the other approaches and has a greater risk of recurrence because the facial nerve is situated between the surgeon and the tumour throughout the dissection and removing tumour that is laterally placed within the internal auditory meatus can be challenging. The likelihood of preserving hearing following hearing preservation surgery is in the region of 50%. All types of surgery have risks of facial nerve injury (risk is related to tumour size and ranges from 2–40%), CSF leak (around 5–10%), Stroke (1–2%), intracranial infection including meningitis (3%), intracranial bleeding (1%), lower cranial nerve injury and death (<1 in 500). Recurrence rates following macroscopic total removal are 1–2%.

3. Radiotherapy: This is an increasingly popular choice, particularly in the older age group. There are 2 main types, stereotactic radiosurgery (SRS) and fractionated radiotherapy. Most centres offer SRS. There are several ways by which SRS can be delivered. The most common are via a Gamma Knife machine or using a linear accelerator (LINAC). The source of radiation is different between these modalities but the outcomes are very similar. The treatment is usually given as a single dose of radiation (usually 14 Gray), although it may be fractionated, and is an out patient procedure with very few early complications. There is an approximately 5% chance of temporary facial weakness during the first few weeks following treatment. The permananent facial palsy rate is around 1%. Longer term there is a slightly higher risk of stroke and a very small risk that the tumour may undergo malignant change. These risks increase with the number of years post-treatment and some centres are reluctant to offer radiotherapy to younger patients for this reason. The radiotherapy does not remove the tumour but is successful in stabilising the tumour in around 95% of cases. The 5% that fail generally require surgical excision and surgery following radiotherapy can be more challenging with poorer facial nerve preservation rates.

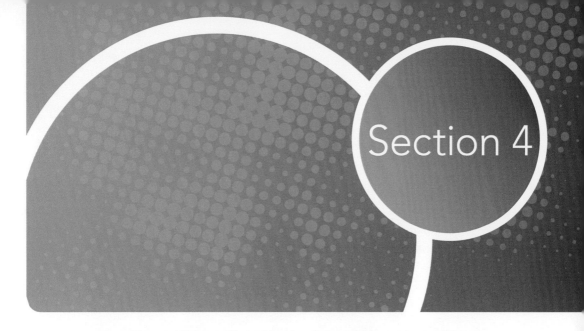

RHINOLOGY AND FACIAL PLASTICS

CASE 50

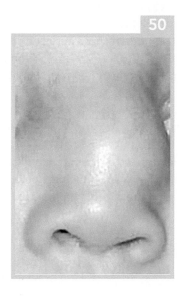

The parents of a 12-month-old baby come to the clinic because of a midline swelling on their son's nose. He is asymptomatic.

i.   What is the likely diagnosis and pathogenesis?

ii.   What is the differential diagnosis?

iii.   How would you investigate this condition?

iv.   How is this condition treated?

i. This is a nasal dermoid. It is a congenital epithelial lined cavity or sinus tract containing variable numbers of skin appendages. It is usually located on the dorsum of the nose between the glabella and columella and may have an intracranial extension.

The pathogenesis can be explained by the widely accepted prenasal space theory. During normal development, a projection of dura protrudes through the fonticulus frontalis (a potential space between the frontal and nasal bones) or inferiorly into the prenasal space. This projection normally regresses but, if it does not, the dura can remain attached to the epidermis and result in trapped ectodermal elements.

ii. Midline congenital nasal lesions are rare: 1/20,000–40,000 births.

The most commonly encountered masses are nasal dermoids, encephaloceles and gliomas. The differential diagnosis also includes epidermoid cysts, haemangiomas, teratomas, neurofibromas, lipomas and lymphatic malformations.

iii. Computed tomography (CT) and magnetic resonance imaging (MRI) scans are the gold standards in radiographic evaluation of nasal dermoids.

CT imaging is useful for visualising bony defects of the skull base and may show findings consistent with intracranial involvement such as an enlarged foramen cecum or bifid crista galli. MRI is more sensitive and specific; it is superior for visualising soft tissues and diagnosing intracranial extension. A biopsy should not be performed before an intracranial connection is ruled out because of the risk of causing meningitis or cerebrospinal fluid (CSF) leak.

iv. Treatment of a nasal dermoid is complete surgical excision of the cyst and any sinus tract. Recurrence rates of 50%–100% have been reported in cases in which dermal components were incompletely removed. The nasal portion of the dermoid can be removed using any one of various incisions, including midline vertical, transverse, lateral rhinotomy, or midbrow or an external rhinoplasty approach. If there is intracranial extension, a neurosurgical evaluation is required and craniotomy is generally performed as part of the procedure. More recently, intranasal endoscopic approaches have been used to resect nasal dermoid cysts including their removal from the dura.

CASE 51

A 70-year-old male has had a basal cell carcinoma excised from his nose.

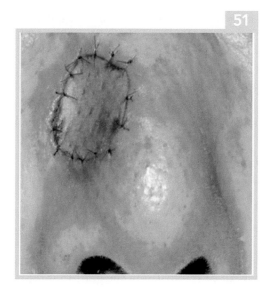

i. What sort of reconstruction has been used?

ii. What are the stages of healing for this type of reconstruction?

iii. What is the failure rate for this method of reconstruction and what are the causes?

Answers 51

i.   It shows that a full-thickness skin graft has been used for reconstruction.

ii.   The first stage is imbibition, whereby simple diffusion keeps the graft from failing. This lasts up to 48 hours.

       The second stage is inosculation, where small capillaries of the donor site become in line with the graft capillaries to allow blood flow. This may last up to 1 week after grafting.

       The third stage is revascularisation, where new vessels are formed to the graft.

iii.   The rate of graft failure for full-thickness skin graft is ~10%–15%.

       There are local and general factors for graft failure.

       Local factors

       Haematoma or infection is the most common. Others include surgical error applying the graft the wrong way round (dermis side down), too much tension on graft, placement on an incorrect tissue bed (i.e. bone, cartilage), failing to immobilise the graft or traumatising the graft (poor surgical technique and handling). Applying a graft to an area of irradiated tissue is less likely to be successful.

       General factors

       Any underlying condition that can cause either haematoma or infection will increase the chance of failure (i.e. aspirin use, diabetes mellitus). Any impairment of healing will increase the chance of failure (vitamin deficiencies, diabetes mellitus, smoking).

QUESTIONS 52

A 50-year-old male patient is referred to clinic with a long-standing history of sneezing and rhinorrohea made worse after eating or drinking. Anterior rhinoscopy shows the following appearance of his left nostril.

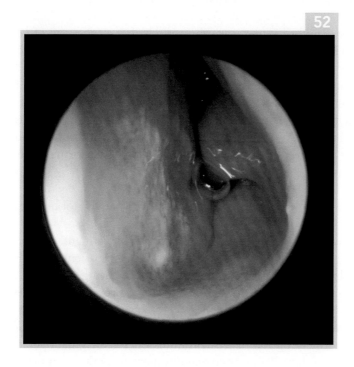

52

i.   What questions are pertinent to ask in the history?

ii.   What is the likely diagnosis?

iii.   What treatment options are you aware of and what are the side effects of those treatments?

i.   Duration of symptoms, when it occurs (perennial vs. seasonal), relation to eating/drinking, relation to certain environments (i.e. around animals), the colour of the nasal discharge, unilateral versus bilateral nasal discharge (do not forget potential cerebrospinal fluid [CSF] leak), any bleeding/bloody discharge (e.g. in tumours), other nasal symptoms of obstruction, smell disturbance, facial pain, post-nasal drip and any trauma or surgery to the nose.

ii. The likely diagnosis is gustatory rhinitis which is a subgroup of non-allergic rhinitis. This is thought to be due to stimulation of the trigeminal nerve in the upper aerodigestive tract (usually in response to spicy foods), which causes a corresponding increase in parasympathetic nerve activity to the nasal mucosa (similar in nature to Frey syndrome). There are four identified subtypes of gustatory rhinitis: idiopathic, post-traumatic, post-surgery and gustatory rhinitis associated with cranial nerve palsies. There is no diagnostic test but often allergy tests (skin prick tests/Radioallergosorbent test) are performed to help exclude allergic rhinitis.

iii. Avoidance of the trigger should be considered (usually not practical).

     Ipratropium bromide nasal spray is the first-line treatment. Its side effects include a dry nose and it can potentially cause problems in patients with glaucoma and prostatic hypertrophy. It should be used prior to eating. Its use in combination with a nasally inhaled corticosteroid appears to provide the best response.

     Vidian neurectomy has been used since the 1960s (described by Golding-Wood) and is a treatment option in recalcitrant cases. The original operation was carried via a Caldwell-Luc approach but more recently it has been carried out endonasally. The risks with this surgery are the same as for standard endoscopic sinus surgery (bleeding, infection, risk to the eye and CSF leak) in addition to the risk of a dry eye (reported at 12%–30%), nasal dryness and crusting.

     More novel treatments include topical capsaicin (an extract from chilli) and botulinum toxin A. There are limited data available as to the long-term success of either of these treatments.

CASE 53

QUESTIONS 53

A 30-year-old man has been referred by the endocrinologist with chronic rhinosinusitis. He also has infertility and chest disease.

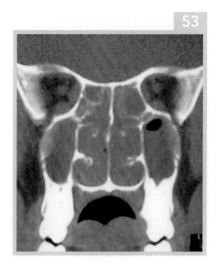

i.   What does his computed tomography (CT) scan of his sinuses show?

ii.   What is the possible diagnosis and what investigations may be useful?

iii.   Describe this condition.

iv.   What treatment as an ENT surgeon can you offer these patients?

Answers 53

i. The coronal CT scan shows a pansinusitis.

ii. The likely diagnosis here is primary ciliary dyskinesis (PCD).

Screening tests for PCD include the following:
- The saccharin test: saccharin is placed approximately 1 cm behind anterior end of inferior turbinate and, if it takes longer than 30 minutes for the patient to taste it, then the test is suggestive of PCD.
- Measuring nasal nitric oxide levels. In PCD, it is lower than in the general population.
- The gold standard test is nasal mucosal biopsy to assess for ciliary ultrastructure in specialised centres.

iii. It is a rare autosomal recessive genetic disorder whereby cilial motility is impaired. Previously it was thought that the cilia were completely immotile but in most cases they do have movement but the movement is inefficient. Therefore, any organ with cilia will be affected, for example the lungs, the nose and paranasal sinuses, the middle ear, sperm in males (the flagella of the sperm) or the fallopian tubes in females. Kartagener's syndrome is a form of PCD that consists of situs inversus, bronchiectasis and chronic rhinosinusitis. Approximately 50% of PCD suffers have this syndrome.

iv. Hearing aids for glue ear should be tried first as grommets tend to be problematic due to persistent discharge and a high rate of tympanic membrane perforation. Medical treatment of chronic rhinosinusitis is with nasal douching and nasal steroids. There is little evidence to support the use of functional endoscopic sinus surgery.

CASE 54

A 13-year-old girl is referred to the clinic because of the appearance of her ears.

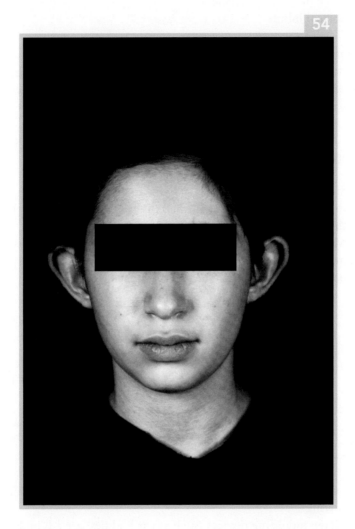

i.   What does the image show?

ii. What are the anatomical abnormalities that contribute to this deformity?

iii. Describe two techniques that might be used to correct this problem?

iv. What are the advantages and disadvantages of both techniques?

v.   Are you aware of any current guidelines regarding management of this condition?

Answers 54

i.   This is a clinical picture of prominent or protruding ears.

ii.   • Deep conchal bowl
        • Absence of the anti-helical fold
        • Abnormal lobule

        The normal size of the ear is 5–6 cm long and its normal orientation is 20° from the vertical plane. The ear should diverge from the scalp at no greater than 35°. The angle between the conchal bowl/scaphoid fossa and anti-helical rim should be between 75° and 105°.

iii.   There are several techniques described for dealing with prominent ears. Two of the more commonly used techniques are:

        1.   Stenstrom technique: The lateral skin and perichondrium is elevated and the lateral surface of the antihelix is abraded causing it to bend away from the abraded side (Gibson's principle)
        2.   Mustarde technique: A portion of post-auricular skin is excised and a mattress suture is placed between the pinna and the skull periosteum in order to close the angle between pinna and skull.

iv.

	Advantages	Disadvantages
Mustarde	Less risk of haematoma	Cartilage needs to be more mature Sutures can cut out or become undone requiring revision
Senstrom	Good result with the ear less likely to unfold and return to the original shape	Haematoma Risk of thermal damage to the lateral part of the ear leading to scarring

v.   A commissioning guide from the Royal College of Surgeons England 2013 states the following:
        • Cartilage moulding devices (such as ear buddies) are advised in infants up to the age of 6 months.
        • Surgery for children with prominent ears should be available on the National Health Service (NHS).
        • Psychological distress in children and adolescents with prominent ears is significant and corrective surgery can help resolve these issues.
        • It is recommended that surgery is only offered to children between the ages of 5 and 18. Children under the age of 5 are less likely to tolerate the procedure

or be compliant with the dressing. Psychological distress is less likely to develop prior to the age of 5 and the surgery can therefore be delayed.

- Surgery should only be offered before the age of 5 if correction of the prominence will help retain hearing aids securely, if these devices are needed.
- NHS surgery for prominent ears should not be offered to adults over the age of 18.

QUESTIONS 55

A patient comes to the clinic having had a previous septoplasty. Anterior rhinoscopy shows a straight septum yet he still complains of a blocked nose.

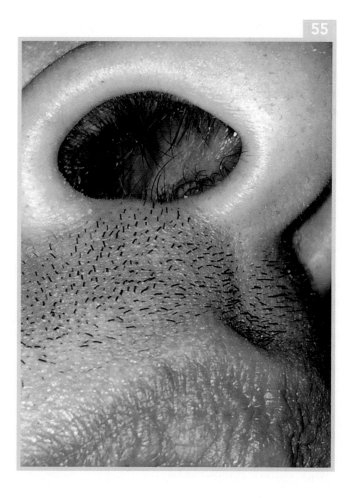

i.   How do you proceed?

ii. What objective tests of nasal patency do you know of?

i. It is important to take a detailed history. This should include:
    - Onset of blockage
    - Timing and side of blockage
    - Precipitating event
    - Alleviating or exacerbating factors
    - Associated nasal symptoms such as anterior rhinorrhoea, postnasal drip, hyposmia, nasal itch, sneezing or epistaxis
    - Any relevant allergies especially to airborne antigens
    - Any treatments and their effectiveness including other operations
    - Any relevant medical conditions eg. asthma, polyangitis with granulomatosis, sarcoidosis
    - Any drug sensitivities eg. to aspirin
    - Any other symptoms such as snoring, weight loss, night sweats

    The patient should then be carefully examined. It is important to assess the nose systematically.
    - The external nose should be assessed for any deformity.
    - The nasal alar should be assessed for significant collapse on deep inhalation
    - The nasal cavity should be examined using a flexible or rigid endoscope to identify any:
        - foreign bodies
        - masses
        - mucosal inflammation
        - crusting
        - The postnasal space should then be assessed for the presence of any obstructive masses.

    The differential diagnosis includes:
    - Foreign bodies
    - Nasal valvular collapse
    - Acute viral rhinosinusitis
    - Acute bacterial rhinosinusitis
    - Allergic chronic rhinosinusitis
    - Non-allergic chronic rhinosinusitis
    - Nasal polyps
    - Benign neoplasia of the nasal cavity eg. inverted papilloma, angiofibroma
    - Malignant neoplasia of the nasal cavity eg. squamous carcinoma, olfactory neuroblastoma
    - Rhinitis medicamentosa
    - Residual adenoidal pad
    - Postnasal space tumours eg. squamous carcinoma
    - Systemic disease eg. sarcoidosis, polyangitis with granulomatosis, tuberculosis

ii.   Misting of a cold metal spatula can provide some information on the patency of
      the nostrils, but no real objective information on airflow.

      Peak nasal inspiratory flow: Peak nasal inspiratory flow (PNIF) is an inexpensive,
      fast, simple technique with excellent reproducibility. It provides a direct measure
      of nasal patency. It utilises a modified Wright peak flow meter with a mask that
      is placed over the patients' nose. They are then asked to inhale as quickly as
      they can with the mouth closed from full expiration. It should be carried out
      standing. Normal male PNIF is between 100 and 150 L/min. Normal female
      PNIF is between 80 and 120 L/min.

      Acoustic rhinometry: Acoustic rhinometry is a reliable means of measuring the
      volume of the nasal cavity. A probe is placed in the nostril and this generates an
      acoustic signal that is reflected from the nasal cavity to provide an assessment of
      cross-sectional area over distance. This is presented as an area–distance curve that
      normally has 3 notches representing the most narrow areas of the nasal cavity.
      The first two are the nasal valve and the front of the inferior turbinate. The third
      is variable. One of these represents the minimum cross-sectional area (MCA).
      The MCA in adults is usually between 1.3 and 1.5 cm^2.

      Rhinomanometry: Rhinomanometry provides a quantitative measure of nasal
      resistance. Active anterior rhinomanometry is the most widely used technique.
      The pressure gradient required to obtain a specific nasal airflow is measured and
      from that nasal resistance is calculated. The pressure gradient is usually fixed at
      150 Pascals. The patient breathes through one nasal cavity whilst the pressure
      difference between nares and choana is measured in the other nasal cavity.
      Normal nasal resistance in adults is 0.25 Pa/cm^3/s.

CASE 56

QUESTIONS 56

A 62-year-old gentleman with a long-standing history of a weak voice is attending the voice clinic for an injection of the following drug.

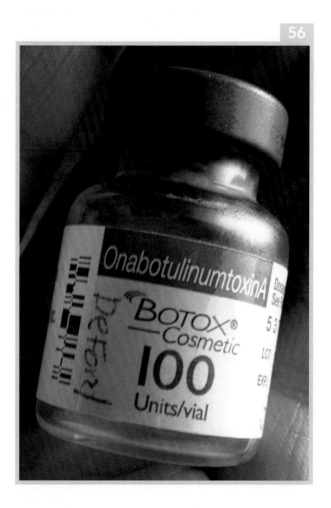

i.   What is botulinum toxin?

ii.   What ENT indications are you aware of for the use of botulinum toxin?

i. Botulinum toxin is a neurotoxin released by *Clostridium botulinum* and prevents release of the neurotransmitter acetylcholine from axons at the neuromuscular junction. It therefore results in flaccid paralysis of skeletal muscle, smooth muscle and the secretion of some glands. It is used clinically to either paralyse muscles (that may be overactive) or reduce secretions from glands. There are various types, A to G with types A and B most commonly used in medical practice.

ii. Frey syndrome: This is caused secondary to parotid surgery whereby eating/ thinking of eating causes sweating and erythema of the skin overlying the parotid gland. This is due to aberrant parasympathetic reinnervation of the skin sweat glands from the dissected parotid gland. Botulinum toxin can be injected into the affected area to paralyse this affect.

Spasmodic dysphonia: This can be for either adduction or abduction spasmodic dysphonia. The type of dysphonia dictates which muscles of the larynx are injected to reduce their activity.

Blepharospasm, torticollis and hemifacial spasm can be treated with botulinum toxin, but are often managed by neurologists.

It may also be used to relax the cricopharyngeus muscle in patients with dysphagia due to cricopharyngeal spasm and in post-laryngectomy patients who have pharyngo-oesophageal spasm resulting in failure of tracheo-oesophageal speech.

Sialorrhoea in those with Parkinson's disease or with cerebral palsy can be treated with botulinum toxin as can palatal and stapedial myoclonus.

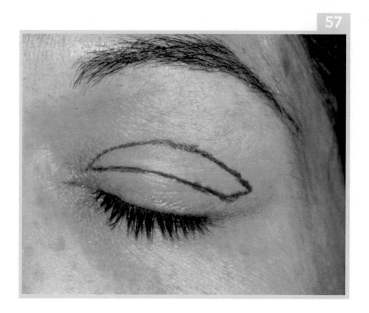

i. What procedure does this picture demonstrate?

ii. What are the indications for this procedure?

iii. What complications can arise as a result of surgery?

Answers 57

i. This image demonstrates the incision made when carrying out an upper lid blepharoplasty.

ii. Functional problems resulting in lid ptosis (defined as covering of >2 mm of the limbus by the upper eyelid):
  - Congenital weakness of the lid
  - Acquired weakness
    - Neurogenic: occulomotor palsy, Horner syndrome, facial nerve palsy
    - Myogenic: myasthenia gravis, myotonic dystrophy, ocular myopathy
    - Aponeurotic: involutional or post-trauma
    - Mechanical: oedema, tumours of the upper lid
    - Pseudotosis: empty socket, atrophic globe, higher lid position on the contralateral side

  Cosmesis

iii. Complications include the following:
  - Retrobulbar haemorrhage when excising orbital fat with loss of vision
  - Ectropion is the most common complication of lower lid blepharoplasty
  - Milia, small subepidermal keratin cysts
  - Lagophthalmos
  - Infection

CASE 58

QUESTIONS 58

A 59-year-old man presents with the following recurrent lesion on the nose following previous primary excision.

The previous histology demonstrates a high-grade morpheaform basal cell carcinoma (BCC). He is discussed at the skin multidisciplinary team (MDT).

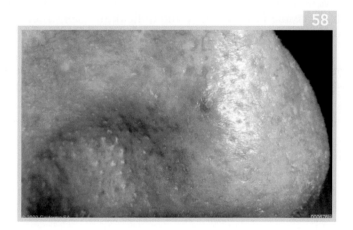

i.   What is the most suitable method of revision surgery given the above history and findings?

ii. Can you describe the principles involved in the procedure?

i. This is a high-risk lesion and the most suitable surgical option would be Mohs micrographic surgery (MMS). The acknowledged indications for the use of MMS are for high-risk cutaneous malignancies or locations:
   - Recurrent or previously incompletely excised cutaneous malignancy
   - High-grade cutaneous malignancy (>2 cm, perineural or perivascular invasion, morpheaform BCC)
   - Indistinct margins clinically (micronodular BCC)
   - High-risk location with high risk of recurrence (i.e. T-zone on face)
   - Area that is cosmetically sensitive and difficult to reconstruct (i.e. nasal alar rim, eyelid)

   Advantages of MMS include the lowest recurrence rate of all treatment modalities, low complication rate, the ability to undertake immediate primary reconstruction. Disadvantages of MMS include difficulty dealing with tumours with skip or satellite lesions, which may be missed on mapping, and difficulties dealing with certain neoplasms, which are sub-optimally assessed using frozen section histology, such as those requiring immunohistochemistry.

ii. MMS is a surgical technique used for the excision of both melanomatous and non-melanomatous skin cancer of the head and neck.

   The technique aims to achieve histologically clear margins, while minimising healthy tissue loss and the functional or cosmetic defect. Studies have shown recurrence rates lower to other surgical modalities, such as wide local excision.

   Cutaneous neoplasms spread both outward and downward from the site of origin. In some cases, deep tumour extension may not be evident from the surface, thus compromising primary wide local excision margins.

   The principle of MMS is that the tumour is mapped, usually into quadrants. During tumour excision, serial sections from each quadrant are excised and assessed microscopically using frozen section histology creating a tumour map and allowing 360° analysis of the margin. This informs the surgeons as to whether each quadrant is clear of tumour. If not, excision in this quadrant continues until examined sections are clear. If clear, no further surgery is required in that quadrant.

CASE 59

A 22-year-old male presents to Accident and Emergency with a history of bilateral nasal obstruction, purulent anterior rhinorrhoea and right sided frontal headache. For the last 48 hours his right eye and forehead has become increasingly swollen.

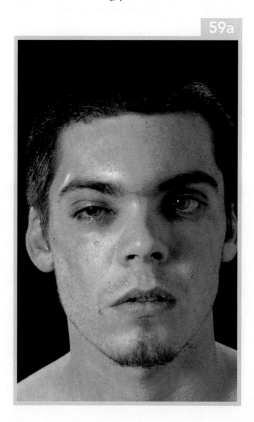

59a

i.   What is the diagnosis?

You see the same patient back in clinic many weeks after his treatment and a recent CT scan shows bilateral frontal sinus complete opacification.

ii.   What important complication can be associated with this condition?

iii. What investigations would you carry out?

iv.   What is the treatment for this condition?

v.   What are the complications that can occur as a result of treatment?

i. This is an osteomyelitis of the right frontal bone with subperiosteal abscess formation. It is also called a Potts puffy tumour although it is not a neoplastic process. The infection originates from the frontal sinus and spreads anteriorly to the frontal bone.

ii. It can be associated with a brain abscess, subdural empyema and cortical vein thrombosis.

iii. A computed tomography (CT) scan of the sinuses and a magentic resonance scan of the head with gadolinium enhancement should be undertaken following a clinical assessment that should include an assessment of conscious level, assessment of visual acuity, colour vision and ocular movements and an endoscopic examination of the nose. The MRI scan for this case is shown below.

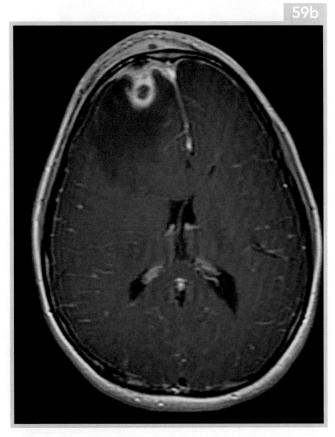

Axial T1 weighted MRI of the head with gadolinium enhancement showing a right frontal lobe abscess with surrounding oedema of the brain

iv.   Medical therapy should be maximised and should include topical intranasal steroids, saline nasal douching and antibiotic treatment based on local microbiology advice. Antibiotic therapy is usually required for a period of 6 to 8 weeks. This is not going to cure this patient's infection, however and he will require surgical treatment of the sinus infection and an urgent opinion from the on call neurosurgeon. Acutely, the brain abscess will require drainage by the neurosurgeons and you will need to drain the frontal sinus infection. Drainage of the frontal sinus infection may be undertaken endonasally or externally. The latter is advisable in the acute setting. The frontal sinus requires trephining followed by washout. The trephine can be undertaken through a small brow incision using a mini-trephine set. Alternatively it can be undertaken using a 3 mm diamond drill. A drain should be left in situ.

In the longer run, in order to avoid further problems, the drainage of the frontal sinuses should be maximised by undertaking an endoscopic drainage procedure as described by Draf. The appropriate procedure for bilateral frontal sinus disease is a Draf type III procedure. The interfrontal septum, floor of the frontal sinuses and superior nasal septum are removed as far as the orbits laterally. The lamina papyracea and posterior wall of the frontal sinus are preserved.

v.   These include crusting, infection, bleeding (risk to anterior ethmoid artery), stenosis of opening (up to 50% of cases), risk to the eye (bruising, bleeding into orbit due to damage of the anterior ethmoid artery, damage to the extra-ocular muscles), risk of cerebrospinal fluid (CSF) leak (due to damage at the first olfactory filia/back wall of frontal sinus) and small risk of nasal collapse due to septal resection.

CASE 60

A 39-year-old man sustains repeated blunt trauma to the face. On examination, he has upper lip swelling, buccal sulcus ecchymosis tenderness, malocclusion and an anterior open bite deformity. Glasgow Coma Scale (GCS) is 15 and he is haemodynamically stable. The reconstructed 3D CT is shown as follows.

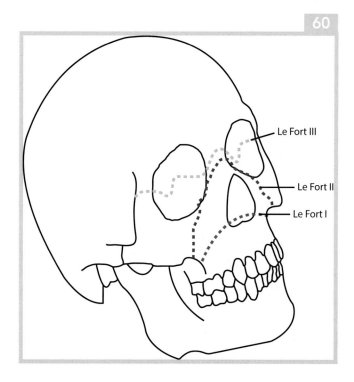

i. What is the diagnosis highlighted by the arrow?

ii. How is this injury classified?

iii. What are the structures at risk in such injuries?

iv. What are the treatment options?

i.   The computed tomography (CT) shows a transverse maxillary fracture, separating the upper alveolus from the upper maxilla. This low maxillary fracture, classified as Le Fort I, extends from the nasal septum to the pyriform aperture, travels above the dental alveolus to below the zygomatic buttress, crossing the pterygomaxillary junctions and interrupting the pterygoid plates.

ii.   The Le Fort classification is used and fractures are classified with respect to highest level of injury. The Le Fort classification has its limitations and it should be noted that injuries may be a combination of two or more types. Furthermore, the degree of force required to sustain such a fracture means that these injuries rarely occur in isolation and are associated with a high incidence of orbital and intracranial injuries. Maxillary fractures may involve injuries not addressed by Le Fort, such as palatal, medial maxillary arch and anterior maxillary fractures.

Le Fort II (pyramidal): It extends from the nasal bridge, at or below the naso frontal suture, passing through the following:
- Frontal process of the maxilla
- Inferolaterally though the lacrimal bones and orbital floor, rim and foramen
- Anterior wall of maxillary sinus
- Under zygoma, pterygomaxillary suture and through the pterygoid plates

Le Fort III (cranial facial dysjunction): These fractures separate the facial skeleton from skull base and require significant force. They pass through the following:
- Nasofrontal suture
- Medial orbital wall, through nasolacrimal groove and ethmoid
- Orbital flow
- Lateral orbital wall
- Zygomatic arch
- Perpendicular plate of ethmoid, internally, vomer and pterygoid plates to the base of sphenoid

iii.   The structures at risk following this type of injury are:
- The infraorbital nerve, which runs through inferior orbital fissure, exiting via the infraorbital foramen. Le Fort fractures II are commonly associated with cheek and upper teeth numbness as this fracture violates the orbital rim.
- The internal maxillary artery branches
- Orbital contents:
  - Globe
  - Optic nerve
  - Lacrimal system
  - Extra ocular muscles

This type of injury is also associated with cerebrospinal fluid leak if there is disruption of the skull base.

iv. Prior to addressing the fracture, all patients should be assessed according to Advanced Trauma and Life Support guidelines. A secure airway must be ensured and any intracranial and C-spine injuries addressed.

Surgical options include the following:
- Maxillary-mandibular fixation (MMF): only recommended for stable, non-displaced Le Fort I
- Open reduction, internal fixation (ORIF): usually undertaken with plating
- External fixation is rarely used in current practice

The goals of treatment are as follows:
- Re-establish midfacial height and width
- Address malocclusion
- Restore soft-tissue contours

CASE 61

QUESTIONS 61

A 45-year-old man with a history of previous nasal surgery complains of intermittent crusting and a whistling noise from his nose.

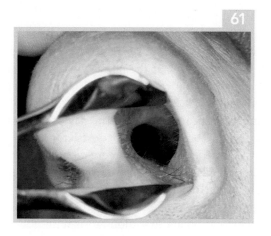

i.   What does the picture show?

ii. What are the causes?

iii. What investigations would you request?

iv. What are the management options?

i. This shows a medium sized nasal septal perforation. It is not possible to see the nasal dorsum in this picture but large perforations may result in an external saddle deformity. The turbulent airflow that results from the septal perforation causes dryness and crusting around the perforation as well as whistling when breathing through the nose.

ii. Common causes include:
- Iatrogenic: Surgery to the nasal septum may result in septal perforation if there is significant trauma or tears to the adjacent parts of the mucosal flaps on each side of the nose at the point where septal cartilage has been excised. Excessive bilateral cautery of the nasal septum can also result in septal perforation.
- Traumatic: Significant trauma to the nasal septum may result in perforation.
- Cocaine abuse: Cocaine is a vasoconstrictor and regular application of cocaine to the nasal septum (usually for recreational purposes) can result in necrosis of septal cartilage because of constriction of the septal perchondrial blood supply, on which the cartilage relies.
- Autoimmune disease: The most common auto-immune diseases resulting in septal perforation are granulomatosis with polyangiitis (GPA; Previously known as Wegener's granulomatosis) and sarcoidosis.
- Infective: Syphilis and tuberculosis can result in septal perforation.
- Malignancy: Sinonasal malignancies can rarely result in septal perforation eg. T cell lymphoma. If there is irregularity of the margins of the perforation or any other suspicion of tumour then the margins of the perforation should be biopsied.

iii. Investigations include:
- Cytoplasmic anti-neutrophil cytoplasmic antibody (cANCA): To identify the presence of GPA.
- Angiotensin Converting Enzyme (ACE): To identify sarcoidosis.
- Erythrocyte Sedimentary Rate (ESR): This is a general inflammatory marker and may be helpful in diagnosis and monitoring of any inflammatory aetiology.
- Treponemal antibodies: This will identify the presence of syphilis.

iv. Conservative: nasal rinsing, moisturisation (prevent crusting). Reconstruction options: prosthesis (septal button) or surgical repair.

The principles of surgical repair involve using mucosal, mucoperichondrial, and/or mucoperiosteal flaps from the nasal cavity, or with connective tissue autograft, to be interposed between the mucosal flaps. These procedures may be endonasal, endoscopic or open.

CASE 62

QUESTIONS 62

A 37-year-old woman presents with a 3-month history of decreased sense of smell and nasal obstruction. She has noticed in the last 2 weeks that she has started to get double vision on looking upward and numbness of her face.

These are her imaging results.

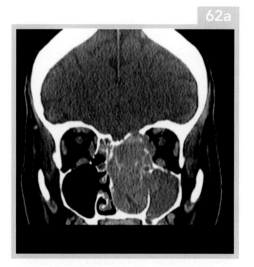

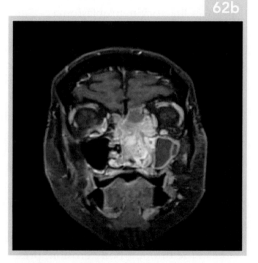

Coronal computed tomography scan of the head with soft tissue windows

Coronal T1 weighted MRI scan of the head with gadolinium enhancement

i.   What is the likely diagnosis in this case? Describe the radiological features that are of concern.

ii. What type of risk factors are associated with this type of pathology?'

iii. How would you manage this patient?

i. The fairly short history and the onset of diplopia suggest that there is an aggressive neoplastic process in this case. Anterior rhinoscopy would demonstrate an obvious polypoid mass in the left nasal cavity. The scans confirm that there is a probable malignancy arising in the left nasal cavity. There is a large unilateral mass with nasal septal destruction, invasion into the left orbit through the lamina papyracea and invasion through the cribriform plate into the anterior cranial fossa. The commonest types of malignant sinonasal tumour are:
    • Squamous cell carcinoma
    • Adenocarcinoma
    • Adenoidcystic carcinoma
    • Olfactory neuroblastoma
    • Esthesioneuroblastoma

ii. Associated risk factors include the following:
    • Hardwood industry for adenocarcinomas
    • Softwood industry for squamous cell carcinoma (SCC)
    • Nickel and chromium workers, shoe and textile workers and those working with hydrocarbons
    • Human papillomavirus (HPV) 16 and 18
    • Epstein–Barr virus (EBV) (lymphomas)

iii. A structured management approach to these patients would include the following:
    • A staging CT scan of the skull base to diaphragm to help determine size of the tumour, bony erosion, presence of cervical disease and distant metastasis.
    • MRI scan of the sinuses, orbit and brain to determine actual size of tumour and differentiate surrounding oedema and mucosal disease. Critical areas include cribiform plate and intracranial extension, orbital, pterygopalatine fossa, sphenoid and frontal sinus involvement.
    • Specific tests: Bence Jones protein for multiple myloma, urinary catacholamines for esthesioneuroblatoma.
    • Biopsy.
    • Fine needle aspiration (FNA) of any neck nodes.
    • Discussion of results at a dedicated multidisciplinary meeting (radiologist, histopathologist, rhinologist, neurosurgeon, ocular plastic surgeon) and planning of further treatment which could include: palliative, chemo-radiotherapy and surgery. For potentially curable tumours, surgery is the mainstay of treatment. In a limited number of cases endoscopic resection may be used and guidance on this approach has been set out in the European position paper on endoscopic management of tumours of the nose and paranasal sinuses. An endoscopic approach is associated with lower post-operative morbidity. For larger tumours open resection is usually offered if there is no brain invasion. This may involve craniofacial resection with

or without orbital exenteration depending on the extent of the disease. Radiotherapy has a role in palliation of unresectable tumours, in poor surgical candidates, in patients with recurrence or in those with lymphoreticular tumours. Combined surgery and adjuvent radiotherapy may also be offered in some circumstances, for example, in those with positive surgical margins, perineural spread or cervical metastases. Chemotherapy may also be offered as a palliative treatment in some cases.

QUESTIONS 63

A 35-year-old man presents to clinic with a swelling behind his left ear.

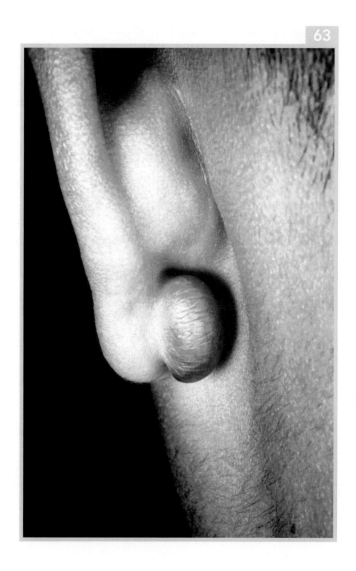

63

i.   What does the picture show and what are the risk factors associated with it?

ii.   What are the phases of wound healing?

i.   Keloid scar: This is a keloid scar of the lobule of the left pinna. Keloids are seen with greater frequency in afrocaribbean, hispanic and asian populations. The most common sites of keloid formation in the head and neck are the earlobes, mandibular border and posterior neck. It results from abnormal proliferation of fibous tissue that forms at the site of cutaneous injury; it does not regress and grows beyond the original margins of the scar. In contrast, hypertrophic scars do not grow beyond the boundaries of the original wound and may regress over time.

Hypertrophic scars and keloids are part of a spectrum of fibroproliferative disorders. They result from the loss of the control mechanisms that normally regulate tissue repair and regeneration.

ii.   The phases of wound healing are as follows:

Inflammatory phase: clot formation followed by phagocytic cells (neutrophils and macrophages)

Proliferation phase: granulation tissue, angiogenesis followed by epithelialisation

Maturation phase: remodelling of collagen from type III to type I

CASE 64

QUESTIONS 64

A 79-year-old gentleman presents to your clinic with a lesion on his nose which bleeds occasionally.

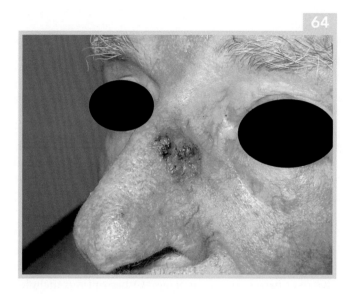

i.   What does the image show?

ii.   What is the likely diagnosis?

iii.   What are the risk factors for this?

iv.   How would you manage this patient?

v.   What are the surgical reconstruction options for this patient?

Answers 64

i. The patient has an irregular erythematous plaque with some scabbing and crusting on the skin of the left nasal dorsum.

ii. It is very suspicious of a cutaneous squamous cell carcinoma. Basal cell carcinoma is also within the differential diagnosis.

iii. Risk factors include:
- Ultraviolet (UV) light
- Immunosuppression
- Exposure to ionising radiation or chemical carcinogens
- Human papillomavirus (HPV) infection
- Skin type

iv. Confirm the diagnosis first with a biopsy of the lesion. Definitive management would include surgical excision with a 4–5 mm margin. This type of lesion would ideally be treated using MOHS surgery. This ensures that the margins of the excision are clear of tumour.

v. Given the size of the lesion and its position, and following the reconstructive ladder, a full-thickness skin graft would be the most appropriate first line of management if there is some soft tissue present on the bed of excision (skin graft does not survive over bare bone or cartilage). Other options include using local flaps. Options might be a forehead flap, a nasolabial flap, a bilobed flap, rhomboid flap or a dorsal nasal rotation flap.

CASE 65

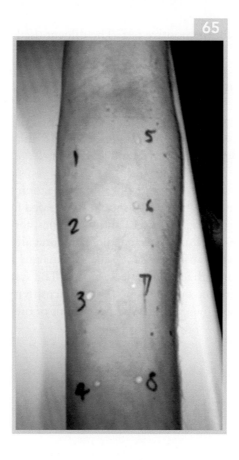

A 34-year-old man presents with a history of persistently blocked and runny nose.

i.   What investigation is being performed?

ii.   What is used for the positive and negative controls?

iii. What skin condition can show a false positive result?

iv.   Which hypersensitivity reaction is occurring and which immunoglobulin is implicated?

v.   What medications can interfere with the results of this investigation?

i. Skin allergy test. There are three types: intradermal test, puncture or prick test and scratch test. This is a skin prick test that is commonly used to identify the common airborne allergens associated with allergic chronic rhinosinusitis including grass and tree pollens, house dust mite and animal fur/dander.

ii. Histamine is used for the positive test. The diluent used for the allergens serves as negative control.

iii. It can be falsely positive in people with dermatographia.

iv. This is a type 1 hypersensitivity – immediate. Mast-cell bound immunoglobulin E (IgE) is implicated. The allergen binds to the IgE and results in degranulation of the mast cell releasing histamine and leukotrienes.

v. Many drugs can interfere with the wheal–flare reaction of the allergy skin test. Therefore, the following drugs should be avoided for the respective time frames before skin testing: H1 or H2 antihistamines, for at least 48 hours; the new antihistamines astemizole, terfenadine and loratadine, for 6 weeks or more; and the tricyclic antidepressants, chlorpromazine hydrochloride and the benzodiazepine tranquilizers, for at least 5 days. The systemic glucocorticoids, which interfere with the delayed type IV hypersensitivity reaction, do not hinder the immediate type I hypersensitivity mechanism of the allergy skin test.

CASE 66

A 16-year-old male presents to the emergency department with a brisk right-sided epistaxis. There is no preceding history of trauma or recent infections. He has noticed that he has had difficulty breathing from the same side over the last 4 months.

When you arrive in casualty, the patient is haemodynamically stable and no longer bleeding. Routine bloods for full blood count (FBC), clotting and urea and electrolytes (U&E) have been sent and come back normal. You examine his nose with a rigid nasendoscope and see a lesion in the right nasal cavity. You organise a magnetic resonance imaging (MRI) scan and computed tomography (CT) scan which are shown as follows.

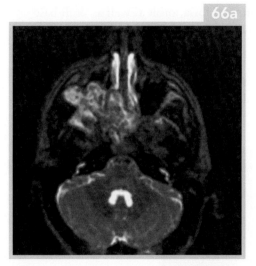

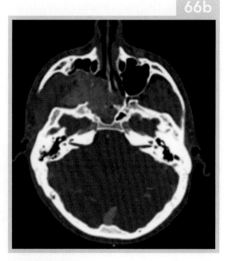

Axial T2-weighted MRI scan of the head

Axial CT scan of the head

i.   What is the likely diagnosis?

ii.   Is there any other imaging you could perform to confirm your suspicion?

iii.   What else could it be?

iv.   How do you stage this pathology?

v.   What are the management options?

i.   In a young man presenting with a unilateral epistaxis with nasal obstruction and a mass arising from the lateral nasal wall in the region of the sphenopalatine artery the likely diagnosis is juvenile nasopharyngeal angiofibroma (JNA). This is confirmed on the imaging, which shows a heterogeneous mass arising from the posterior lateral nasal wall, enlarging the sphenopalatine foramen and extending into the infratemporal fossa. These are benign lesions accounting for 0.05% of head and neck tumours. They occur exclusively in males predominantly in the second decade with the highest incidence between the ages of 7 and 19 years. They rarely occur over the age of 25. CT scans can help to demonstrate bony involvement of the paranasal sinuses, orbit, pterygomaxillary fossa, greater wing of the sphenoid, basesphenoid and baseocciput. MRI scan allows for more accurate assessment of the size of the lesion and extent of expansion into the pterygomaxillary fossa/infratemporal fossa, orbit as well as skull base and intracranial spread. Biopsy is not advocated as this would cause brisk haemorrhage.

ii.   Yes. An angiogram shows a vascular blush on contrast injection. A typical example is shown below. Cross-sectional angiography may also be helpful.

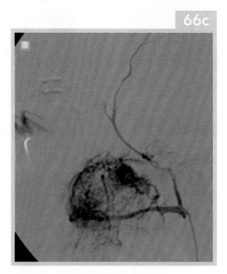

Catheter angiogram of the internal maxillary artery demonstrating a vascular blush on injection of contrast consistent with a JNA.

iii.   The differential diagnosis would include the following:

Inflammatory	Neoplastic (Benign)	Neoplastic (Malignant)	Congenital
Nasal polyps	Inverted papilloma	Rhabdomyosarcoma	Encephalocele
Antrochoanal polyp	–	Squamous cell carcinoma	Teratoma
–	–	Esthesioneuroblastoma	Dermoid
–	–	Melanoma	–

iv.   There are two classification systems.

Classification according to Sessions

Staging	Description
Stage IA	Tumour limited to posterior nares and/or nasopharyngeal vault
Stage IB	Tumour involving posterior nares and/or nasopharyngeal vault with involvement of at least one paranasal sinus
Stage IIA	Minimal lateral extension into pterygomaxillary fossa
Stage IIB	Full occupation of pterygomaxillary fossa with or without superior erosion of orbital bones
Stage IIIA	Erosion of skull base (i.e. middle cranial fossa/pterygoid base); minimal intracranial extension
Stage IIIB	Extensive intracranial extension with or without extension into cavernous sinus

Radowski's classification

Staging	Description
I (A)	Limited to posterior nares and/or nasopharyngeal vault
I (B)	Involving the posterior nares and/or nasopharyngeal vault with involvement of at least one paranasal sinus
II (A)	Minimal lateral extension into the pterygopalatine fossa
(B)	Full occupation of pterygopalatine fossa with or without superior erosion orbital bones
(C)	Extension into the infratemporal fossa or extension posterior to the pterygoid plates
III (A)	Erosion of skull base (middle cranial fossa/base of pterygoids) – minimal intracranial extension
(B)	Extensive intracranial extension with or without extension into the cavernous sinus

v.   Surgery, radiotherapy and medical therapy have all been used to treat JNA.

Surgery

Open surgical resection has historically been the mainstay of treatment although increasingly, endoscopic approaches have been used for tumours as large as Radkowski stage IIIa. Open approaches include transpalatal, lateral rhinotomy and midfacial degloving techniques. Endoscopic resection has the advantage of less bleeding, less morbidity, shorter hospital stay and similar recurrence rates to open surgery. Endoscopic resection does, however, become challenging in tumours with lateral invasion of the infratemporal fossa. Combined endoscopic and open approaches may be used in some cases. Guidance regarding endoscopic approaches has been provided in the European position paper on endoscopic management of tumour of the nase and paranasal sinuses. All surgery should be preceded with embolisation of the feeding vessels 24 to 48 hours pre-operatively. Recurrence tends to occur at the basi-sphenoid, particularly around the Vidian canal and this region should be drilled out to minimise recurrence risk.

Radiotherapy

Radiotherapy, in the form of external beam or intensity modulated radiotherapy, may be offered for unresectable tumours, cases of incomplete tumour resection, for those with extensive intracranial involvement and in those with recurrent tumours. Considerable long term morbidity has, however, been reported, particularly as those treated are often young. Complications include cataract formation, growth impairment, central nervous system syndrome (encephalopathy or dementia) and radiation induced tumours.

Medical Therapy

Hormonal therapy (flutamide, a testosterone receptor blocker) has been used in some centres although its efficacy is unclear and it is not in routine clinical use.

QUESTIONS 67

A 45-year-old man presents to your outpatient department with a history of frequent nose bleeds. He recalls his mother having a similar problem. He has on one occasion been admitted to another ENT department requiring nasal packing and a blood transfusion. You examine the patient and this is what you see.

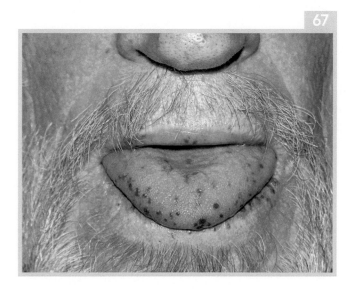

i.   What is the diagnosis?

ii.   What treatment options are available for his epistaxis?

iii.   What other problems might this gentleman experience?

i. This is a clinical picture demonstrating multiple telangectasia affecting the oral mucosa and face in keeping with hereditary haemorrhagic telangiectasia (HHT) (Osler–Weber–Rendu syndrome).

ii. Therapeutic options for HHT-related epistaxis vary from conservative to aggressive surgical treatments. Patients present with varying degrees of severity and treatment is best tailored to the individual patient. The following are the treatment options:

Prophylatic procedures

- Medical therapy: Using oral oestrogen with tamoxifen or topical oestrogen or aminocaproic acid, an anti-fibrinolytic agent
- Sequential laser therapy: Using an argon or KTP laser
- Septodermoplasty: Replacement of the nasal septal mucosa with squamous epithelium
- Surgical closure of the nasal cavity (Young's procedure)

Active bleeding

Avoid packing the nose if possible as this may cause further mucosal trauma. If packing is required, aim to use ribbon gauze soaked in adrenaline, Surgicel or Kaltostat.

Patients in both groups may need blood transfusion.

iii. Besides telangiectasia involving the skin and mucous membranes there may be arteriovenous malformations involving the liver and lungs, gastrointestinal bleeds and arteriovenous malformation in the central nervous system.

CASE 68

QUESTIONS 68

A 42-year-old patient presents with left-sided nasal obstruction with intermittent epistaxis. The following image demonstrates an endoscopic view of the nasal cavity. The contralateral nasal cavity is normal.

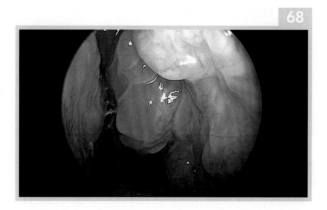

i.   How would you investigate this patient?

ii. A biopsy shows it to be an inverted papilloma. What percentage of inverted papillomas becomes malignant?

iii. How would you treat this patient and are there any relevant guidelines you might use?

iv. What are the recurrence rates?

i. The first line investigation would be a computed tomography scan of the sinuses and a magnetic resonance scan of the sinuses and brain. A biopsy can then be taken to identify the type of pathology.

ii. Between 5% and 15% of inverted papillomas become malignant with squamous cell carcinoma being the most common. Adenocarcinomas and small cell carcinomas have rarely been reported.

iii. According to the guidelines from the European position paper on endoscopic management of nasal tumours 2010, the mainstay of treatment of inverted papillomas is adequate surgical removal of all diseased mucosa and mucoperiosteum.

All patients with these tumours should be managed in a multidisciplinary setting.

Traditional surgical approaches such as lateral rhinotomy, Caldwell Luc and midface degloving have been superseded by the rapid development of endoscopic surgery. Superior imaging and angled instruments and scopes have allowed access into the floor and anterior wall of the maxillary sinus. Median drainage procedures of the frontal sinus have also allowed access into this area. Radiotherapy is not effective against inverted papilloma and is reserved for malignant transformation as an adjunct to surgical therapy or for those who cannot tolerate surgery.

iv. The recurrence rate following endoscopic surgery is similar to open approaches (14.5% vs. 16.7%, respectively) but endoscopic surgery is associated with less morbidity and shorter hospital stays.

QUESTIONS 69

A 45-year-old male attends hospital with a significant epistaxis. Nasal packing is unsuccessful and you take him to theatre.

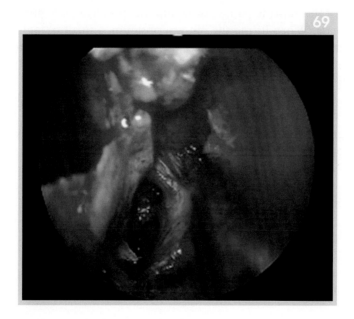

i.   What does this intra-operative image show?

ii.   What are the anatomical landmarks when performing this operation?

iii. Why might this operation be unsuccessful?

i. This is an endoscopic view of a right nasal cavity showing the sphenopalatine artery arising from the sphenopalatine foramen.

ii. The following are helpful anatomical landmarks:
- The sphenopalatine artery arises from the lateral nasal wall (perpendicular plate of the palatine bone) just behind the posterior attachment of the middle turbinate. When lifting the mucoperiosteum, a small triangle of bone called the crista ethmoidalis lies just anterior and superficial to the foramen containing the artery.

iii. The terminal branches of the sphenopalatine artery (SPA) include the following:

a. Septal artery that runs over the face of the sphenoid sinus onto the posterior septal wall.

b. Posterior lateral nasal artery that passes downward over the perpendicular plate of the palatine bone.

It is important to try and identify these branches when performing ligation of the SPA in order to control epistaxis. Failure to ligate both branches may lead to recurrent epistaxis. Ligation is carried out using ligaclips, bipolar or a combination of both.

The sphenopalatine artery supplies the lateral wall of the nose with blood and bleeding from this area is therefore likely to originate from the SPA. Bleeding from other areas of the nasal cavity may originate from other vessels. For example, the anterior and posterior ethmoid arteries supply the bulk of the nasal septum with a contribution from the superior labial artery and the greater palatine artery. The anastomosis of these vessels in Kisselbach's plexus situated in Little's area of the anterior septum is a common source of epistaxis. Bleeding from these areas is unlikely to respond to SPA ligation.

QUESTIONS 70

A 50-year-old gentleman complains of nasal blockage and a whistling noise in his nose.

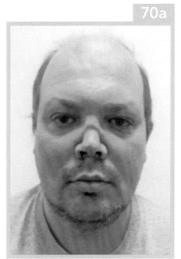

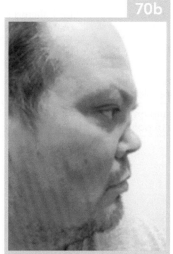

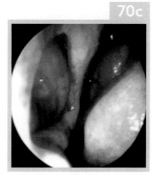

i.   Describe what you see in the images?

ii.   What is your differential diagnosis?

iii.   What is the likely diagnosis?

iv.   List other areas in the head and neck that may be affected?

v.   What tests help with diagnosis?

vi.   How do you treat this condition from a general and ENT point of view?

Answers 70

i. This is a saddle deformity of the nose with an associated septal perforation and generalised chronic rhinosinusitis.

ii. Differential diagnosis

Infective	Inflammatory	Traumatic	Neoplastic
Tuberculosis	Sarcoidosis	Self-inflicted digital trauma	T-cell lymphoma
Leprosy	Churg–Stauss	Iatrogenic	Squamous cell carcinoma
Rhinoscleroma	Eosinophilic granuloma	–	–
Syphilis	Granulomatosis with polyangiitis	–	–
Actinomycosis	–		
Aspergilosis	–		–
Rhinosporidiosis	–		–
Histoplasmosis	–	–	–
Leishmaniasis	–	–	–

iii. Wegener's granulomatosis (WG), now known officially as granulomatosis with polyangiitis (GPA).

iv. ENT manifestations of GPA are common with more than 70% of presenting symptoms involving the upper respiratory tract prior to pulmonary or renal involvement. Head and neck involvement include the following:

Sinonasal manifestation
- Osteocartilagenous destruction manifests as saddle deformity, septal perforation and a painful nasal dorsum.
- Nasal mucosal oedema presents with obstruction, crusting, epistaxis and ulceration. Chronic rhinosinusitis (bacterial and fungal) affects 40%–50% of patients with GPA.

Otological manifestation
- Serous otitis media is the most common presentation (40%–70%) secondary to Eustachian tube obstruction. This can lead to secondary bacterial infection with intervening acute otitis media and mastoiditis.
- Sensorineural hearing loss and vertigo can be due to inflammation of the blood vessels supplying the cochlear, labyrinth or vestibulo-cochlear nerve.

- Similarly vasculitis and granulomas can affect the facial nerve causing facial palsy. Large inflammatory masses in the petrous apex and skull base can also affect cranial nerves VI, IX, XII.

Oropharyngeal manifestations
- Chronic ulceration of the oral mucosa occurs in 6% of patients with GPA. Strawberry gingival hyperplasia is pathogenomic of GPA.
- Inflammation and destruction of the salivary glands.

Laryngotracheal manifestations
- 16%–20% of patients with GPA have subglottic stenosis (50% of paediatric patients).

v. The following tests working in conjunction with each other help with the diagnosis of GPA:

Blood tests
- Routine bloods may show deranged urea and electrolytes (U&E) test with renal involvement, normochromic normacytic anaemia on full blood count (FBC) and raised erythrocyte sedimentation rate (ESR) and C-reactive protein (CRP) during active disease.
- Specific tests include cytoplasmic-antineutrophil cytoplasmic autoantibody (c-ANCA) and perinuclear antineutrophil cytoplasmic antibody (p-ANCA): c-ANCA directed against proteinase 3 (PR3) is most specific for GPA. Using both immunofluoresence and ELISA, cANCA is detectable in nearly 100% of patients with active generalized GPA. Some patients with GPA express p-ANCA specific for myeloperoxidase (MPO). This only occurs in about 13% of patients with active GPA. A positive c-ANCA test result in patients only with sinusitis has a probability of 7%–16% of correctly diagnosing GPA. In patients with sinusitis, pulmonary infiltrates or nodules, and active urinary sediment, a positive c-ANCA test finding has probability of 98% of diagnosing GPA.

Chest x-ray (CXR)
- Findings on chest radiography are abnormal in two thirds of adults with GPA. The most common radiologic findings are single or multiple nodules and masses. Nodules are typically diffuse, and approximately 50% are cavitated.

Tissue biopsy
- The diagnosis of GPA is generally confirmed with tissue biopsy from a site of active disease and renal and lung biopsies are most specific for GPA. Upper respiratory tract tissue biopsies (nose, sinuses, subglottic region) are frequently non-diagnostic, yielding only non-specific acute and chronic inflammation in up to 50% of biopsy samples and demonstrating the full pathologic triad of granulomatous inflammation, vasculitis and necrosis in only about 15% of cases.

Urine analysis
- Protein and red cells casts.

vi.   Treatment would consist of the following:
- Multidisciplinary approach involving rheumatologists, chest and renal physicians. The mainstay of treatment for GPA is a combination of corticosteroids and cytotoxic agents including cyclophosphamide, methotrexate and azathioprine.
- Local treatment:
    - Saline douching and topical steroids for the nose
    - Myringotomy and grommet insertion
    - Hearing aids
    - Reconstructive surgery on the nose only after a full year in remission
    - Subglottic dilatation, tracheostomy and reconstruction

CASE 71

QUESTIONS 71

A patient is referred by the medical team with recurrent meningitis. They had a nasal polypec-tomy 3 years before and since then have been experiencing unilateral nasal discharge. The fol-lowing is a coronal computed tomography (CT) scan of the sinuses taken on admission.

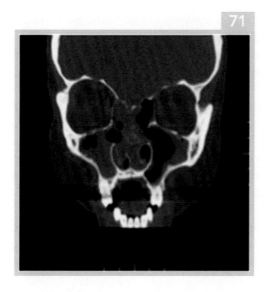

i.   What do you think the problem might be?

ii.   What investigations would you want to perform?

iii.   How would you treat this?

i. It is likely that the patient has a cerebrospinal fluid (CSF) leak as a result of the nasal surgery. The reported risk of CSF leak following nasal polypectomy varies between 0% and 2.3%. A pertinent history should include unilateral clear nasal discharge, salty taste, post-nasal drip and episodes of recurrent meningitis.

ii. *Flexible nasendoscopy.* This can help identify the site of the leak.

   TAU protein (Beta-2 transferrin) on any nasal fluid collected by the patient. The presence of TAU protein is diagnostic of CSF (a serum test for TAU protein if performed helps to increase certainty). There is no modern day role for glucose testing in the investigation of CSF leaks.

   Imaging. High-resolution CT imaging of the skull base is good at identifying the location of leak; however, artefacts can occur (e.g. vessels passing through skull base). The CT is also necessary if navigation-guided surgery is planned. MRI (especially with constructive interference in steady-state [CISS] sequences) can also be useful in identifying the site if there is also a skull base defect such as a meningocele.

   Fluorescein lumbar puncture. This is used as a last resort to help to identify both the presence and site of a leak. There is a small risk of seizure. A concentration of less than 5% is normally used.

iii. This patient requires endoscopic endonasal repair of the CSF leak – the technique depends on the size and site of the leak. There are advocates of single-layer closure, two-layer closure or three-layer closure.

   Free grafts. Mucosa is obtained from inferior turbinate, middle turbinate or temporalis fascia. Ear lobe fat can be used as a bath plug technique. This is useful for small defects. Muscle can also be used (i.e. from thigh). Bone is also used from middle/inferior turbinates as part of a layering technique.

   Pedicled flaps. This can comprise inferior turbinate, nasoseptal flap and galeal flap. It is generally better for larger defects as they have a blood supply.

   Xenogeneic materials. There are a variety of materials that use collagen substituent that can be used either alone or as part of a layered system of closure, for example, DuraGen (Integra LifeSciences Corporation).

QUESTIONS 72

A 13-year old is referred to you by the respiratory team with a history of a blocked nose and recurrent chest infections. Examination reveals bilateral nasal polyps. Their computed tomography (CT) scan is shown as follows.

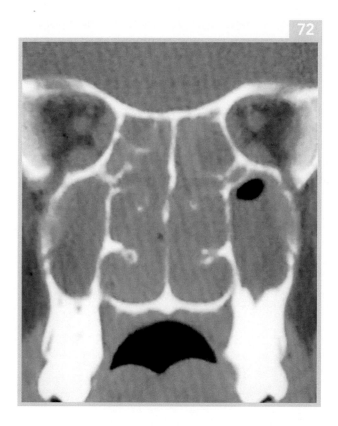

i.   What is the likely underlying diagnosis?

ii.   What is the genetic component of this condition and what diagnostic tests are used?

iii.   Does the treatment of nasal polyps in this condition differ?

i. In this age group, you have to be strongly suspicious of cystic fibrosis (40% of patients with cystic fibrosis have nasal polyps).

ii. Cystic fibrosis is an autosomal recessive condition caused by mutations of the cystic fibrosis transmembrane conductance regulator (*CFTR*) gene on chromosome 7. The defect in this gene leads to altered chloride transport, which affects mucous by making it thicker. This in turn leads to lower and upper respiratory and gastrointestinal tract problems. The sweat test assessing the chloride levels in sweat is the most commonly used test. Genetic testing is also possible to identify the defective gene. Screening for cystic fibrosis in newborns has been available routinely since 2007 based on a heel-prick sample.

iii. The EPOS 2012 guidelines suggest that standard treatment of nasal steroids and douching in addition to endoscopic sinus surgery in failed medical treatment is best. There is some potential benefit in using nasally inhaled dornase alpha and topical antibiotics in chronic rhinosinusitis with polyps. Treating the nasal polyps in patients with cystic fibrosis appears to benefit the lower respiratory tract disease.

CASE 73

A 70-year-old patient attends clinic having been referred from the ophthalmologist with a watery left eye. The opthalmologist has requested some imaging.

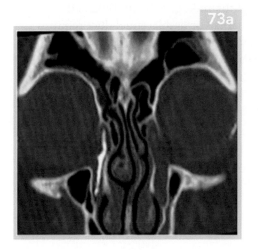

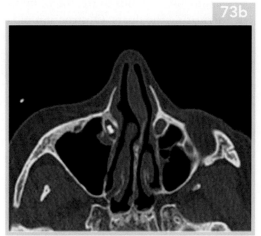

i.   What imaging is this and what does it show?

ii.   What treatment options are available?

iii. Is there any benefit in using a stent?

i.   This is a computed tomography (CT) dacryocystogram. It shows contrast in
      the right nasolacrimal duct and no contrast in the left nasolacrimal duct. This
      suggests a blockage of the left nasolacrimal duct.

ii.   Treatment depends upon where the obstruction is. Obstruction at the
      caniliculi responds to treatment by the ophthalmologists by probing and
      irrigating the ducts. Obstruction of lacrimal sac or nasolacrimal duct requires
      dacrocystorhinostomy (DCR). DCR may be performed via an external or an
      endoscopic approach. The external approach is the standard approach and studies
      have shown success rate of between 80% and 90%. The endoscopic endonasal
      approach has success rates of between 70% and 90%. The main benefit of an
      endonasal approach is the lack of scar. It is also a quicker procedure.

iii. This is controversial. There is evidence to suggest that the success rate is just as
      high in patients without stents. The risks of the stent are possible granulation
      formation at the opening of the DCR, possible slitting of caniliculi and erosion
      of punctum.

A patient has been referred by the ophthalmologist with problems with intermittent eye swelling. You organise some imaging.

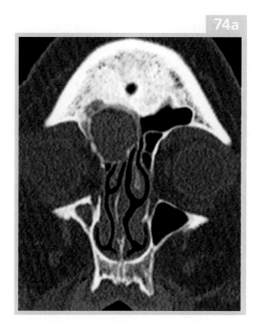

74a

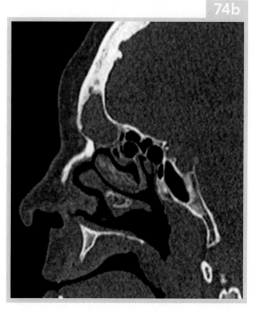

74b

i. What does their computed tomography (CT) scan show and what is the likely diagnosis?

ii. What is the pathogenesis of this condition?

iii. How do you treat this condition and is it likely to recur?

i. The scans show an expansile lesion of the right frontal sinus. It is likely to be a mucocoele. A magnetic resonance imaging (MRI) scan can help with the diagnosis by showing that it is fluid filled, but not cerebrospinal fluid (CSF).

ii. A mucocoele forms as a result of an obstructed sinus, which can be secondary to trauma, surgery, allergy, nasal tumours or it may be congenital. The mucocoele is a mucous filled cyst that is sterile but can get infected and hence cause fluctuation in symptoms as its size changes. The frontal sinus is most likely to be affected.

iii. The mucocoele and sinus pathway need to be opened. In this case, it could be performed by an endoscopic endonasal approach to open the frontal recess on the right side. A Draf 2b procedure (opening the frontal sinus between the lamina papyracea/nasal bone laterally and the nasal septum medially) is most likely to give the best result. Endoscopic endonasal surgery can be considered for disease of the frontal sinus where the pathology does not extend laterally beyond a line in relation to the middle of the pupil of the eye.

Recurrence rates are variable with some studies finding no recurrence whereas others have reported rates up to 23%.

QUESTIONS 75

You are referred a patient who underwent imaging for chronic headaches.

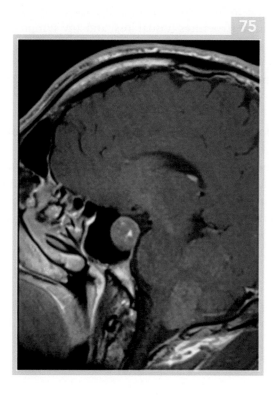

i.   What does this scan show?

ii.   What history would you look for and what investigations would you perform for this patient?

iii.   What tumours are you aware of that cause this?

iv.   When is surgery indicated here?

i.   This is a sagittal computed tomography (CT) image showing a lesion in the pituitary fossa. It is difficult to comment on size, but it is likely to be a macroadenoma.

ii.   Pertinent questions in the history include any symptoms that may be caused by compression of local structures (visual loss) and any symptoms to suggest the tumour is secreting hormones (i.e. Cushing, acromegaly).

Investigations include visual fields and blood tests (pituitary function, electrolytes).

The management of this patient will also require endocrinology input.

iii.   Pituitary tumours are benign or malignant, functioning or non-functioning and symptomatic or non-symptomatic. They are predominantly asymptomatic, benign, non-functioning tumours. The benign varieties are mainly adenomas and are classified as macro or microadenoma based on their size (greater or smaller than 1 cm). The most common functioning benign tumour is the prolactinoma. Other tumours include those causing acromegaly and Cushing disease.

iv.   Surgery is required for non-functioning tumours that threaten vision, acromegaly, Cushing disease and in the patients with failed medical therapy of prolactinomas.

QUESTIONS 76

A 56-year-old man has a history of hayfever and recurrent right-sided sinusitis. He now feels his right cheek appears lower than the left side. You organise some imaging.

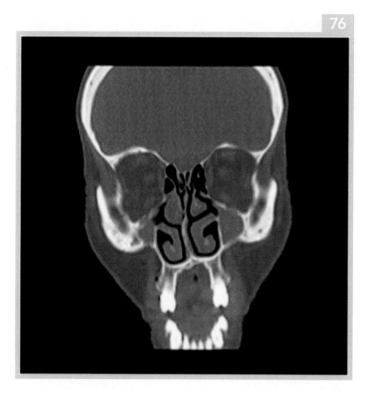

i.   What does this image show and what is the likely diagnosis?

ii. How does this condition present?

iii. How do you treat it?

i. This is a coronal computed tomography (CT) image showing mucosal thickening in both the maxillary sinuses. The most striking feature is that there is asymmetry of the maxillary sinuses, with the right side being smaller than the left and the orbital floor is lower as a result. This raises the possibility of the silent sinus syndrome. This is a condition in which there is spontaneous collapse of the maxillary sinus and orbital floor due to negative pressure within the sinus.

ii. In the majority of patients it is asymptomatic. The most common presenting complaint is that of asymmetry of the cheek. It may also rarely cause diplopia due to enophthalmos.

iii. In the symptomatic patient aeration of the sinus through functional endoscopic sinus surgery, with a middle meatal antrostomy, is beneficial. At a later stage, surgery to address the diplopia and cosmesis can be considered (generally by a maxilla-facial team).

CASE 77

A 50-year-old patient presents with a bilateral blocked nose, reduced smell and nasal discharge. Examination reveals bilateral nasal polyps.

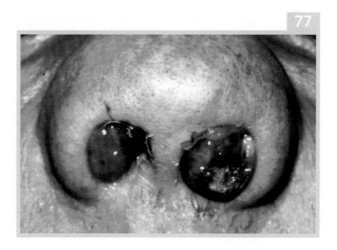

i.   How are you going to treat this patient?

ii.   At what point do you consider surgery for nasal polyps and what operation would you perform?

iii. What other treatments are you aware of for nasal polyps?

i. According to EPOS 2012 guidelines, steroid treatment (either nasally or orally if polyps are completely obstructing nasal cavity) and nasal douching are the most effective treatments. There is some evidence for the use of doxycycline as a 3-week course. There is no evidence for anti-histamines. Arrange follow-up to see if treatment has worked.

ii. Indications for surgery include symptomatic nasal obstruction after medical treatment, more than two courses of oral steroids in a year (according to EPOS 2012) or suspicion of another lesion (i.e. inverted papilloma, malignancy). Operating on polyps due to anosmia is unlikely to be successful in improving their anosmia long term.

The options for operation are either a simple polypectomy or to consider this in addition to endoscopic sinus surgery. There are numerous articles on this but there is no high level of evidence to suggest endoscopic sinus surgery and polypectomy is superior to polypectomy alone.

iii. *Leukotriene antagonists such as montelukast.* This form of treatment is not recommended in the EPOS 2012 guidelines because most of the literature suggests very limited efficacy.

5-Lipoxygenase inhibitors such as zileuton. This is a new treatment for asthma but there is no evidence for use in nasal polyps as yet.

Anti IgE and anti IL-5 treatments are also available and are used in certain groups of patients with asthma. As yet there is no strong data to suggest their use in nasal polyps.

Salicylate avoidance in Samter's triad patients (asthma, nasal polyps and aspirin sensitivity). This is often difficult for patients to achieve due to the large number of foods that contain salicylates and there is no strong evidence for its use in improving nasal polyp symptoms.

Salicylate desensitisation in Samter's triad patients. This can be performed by the oral route (using aspirin) or by the nasal route (using lysine-acetylsalicylate douching). There is good evidence for the oral route but less for nasal desensitisation.

Section 5

PAEDIATRICS

QUESTIONS 78

A 5-year-old boy is brought to hospital at 11 PM because he told his parents that he swallowed something but did not say what it is. He is not in distress and is swallowing his saliva. His chest x-ray is shown below. There is currently a laparotomy in the emergency operating room that will take another 4 hours to finish.

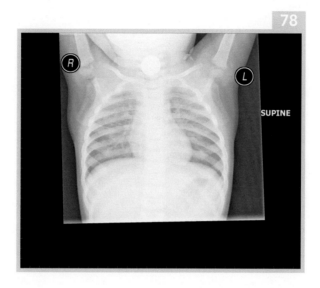

i.   What does the x-ray show?

ii.   What would you do?

Answers 78

i.   The x-ray shows a foreign object just above the level of the clavicles.

ii.   In this case it is unclear what the object is. If you look closely, there is a 'ring' at the edge of the object, which raises the suspicion of a button battery. If this is suspected, it must be treated as a life-threatening case and removed as soon as possible as he is at high risk of perforation and its subsequent sequelae. A second operating room needs to be opened and the operation performed regardless of his fasting time.

CASE 79

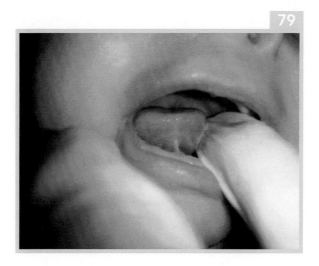

The parents of a 2-month-old baby come to your clinic saying that their child is having difficulty with breast feeding.

i.   What does the image show?

ii. How would you treat this?

i. Tongue tie (ankyloglossia) is a congenital condition where the frenulum is unusually thick, tight or short.

ii. The evidence for the effectiveness of tongue-tie division is variable but overall is considered beneficial, especially if concerns have been raised about feeding. Due to the low morbidity involved with the procedure, it is commonly performed and in some centres without a general anaesthetic.

CASE 80

QUESTIONS 80

A 10-year-old child has a lymphatic malformation excised due to shortness of breath caused by airway compression.

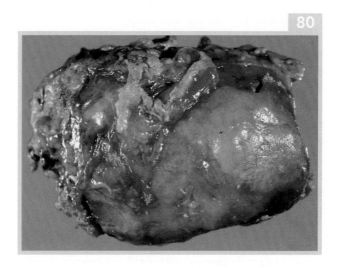

i.   What is a lymphatic malformation?

ii. How are they classified?

iii. How do they classically appear on magnetic resonance imaging (MRI)?

iv. What are the treatment options?

v.   What is OK-432? Are there any other agents that produce a similar effect?

i. A lymphatic malformation is a congenital malformation of the lymphatic system consisting of abnormally dilated endothelially lined lymphatic channels or spaces that result from an embryological error whereby sprouting lymphatics become sequestered during the development of lymphaticovenous sacs. 70% present at birth and 90% have presented by the age of 2 years. 70% present in the head and neck.

ii. They can be classified based on the following:
    • Size:
        • Macrocystic (consisting of cystic space larger than 2 cm²; historically called cystic hygroma)
        • Microcystic (consisting of cystic spaces smaller than 2 cm²; historically called lymphangioma)
    • Location: suggested by Serres et al.
        • Stage I Unilateral infrahyoid
        • Stage II Unilateral suprahyoid
        • Stage III Unilateral infrahyoid and suprahyoid
        • Stage IV Bilateral suprahyoid
        • Stage V Bilateral infrahyoid and suprahyoid

    This classification yields five possible stages that have demonstrated clinical relevance in terms of predicting operative risk and surgical outcome.

iii. It appears as a cystic lesion: hypointense on T1, hyperintense on T2, and may show either no enhancement or rim enhancement with contrast.

    Spontaneous involution is rare and conservative management is rarely acceptable to parents given the cosmetic implications.

iv. Treatment options typically included conservative management, sclerotherapy and surgery. Newer treatments include radiofrequency ablation and laser for small, microcystic and superficial, mucosal-based lesions particularly in the larynx and oral mucosa.

v. OK-432 is a lyophilised mixture of *Streptococcus pyogenes* treated with benzylpenicillin. It works as an immunomodulator, upregulating several cytokines and results in inflammatory response leading to fibrosis + sclerosis. Other sclerosants include ethanol, doxycycline bleomycin, sodium tetradecyl sulphate, acetic acid and hypertonic saline. Sclerotherapy is used for predominantly macrocystic lesions especially if they are surgically challenging.

CASE 81

QUESTIONS 81

The parents of this child attend your clinic complaining that their son persistenly drools.

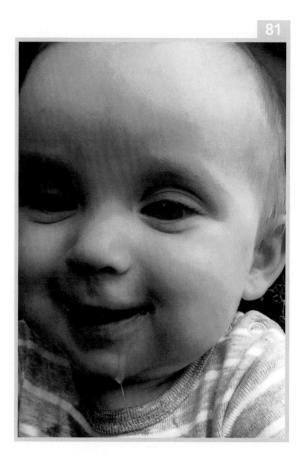

i.   Until what age is this condition normal?

ii.   What are the implications of this condition?

iii. What are the common causes of this condition?

iv.   What are the treatment options?

i. Drooling is normal until the age of 24 months. After 4–5 years of age, it is uniformly considered abnormal.

ii. Medical implications include skin maceration, malodour and, in severe cases, dehydration or aspiration pneumonia. Social implications include frequent bib/clothing changes, less physical contact from parents/caregivers and isolation.

iii. Drooling can be caused by impaired neuromuscular control or, less commonly, hypersecretion. Common causes include cerebral palsy (dysfunctional oral motor control and poor head positioning) and medications such as tranquillisers, anticonvulsants and anticholinesterases.

iv. Treatment options can be classified as medical and surgical:
   - Medical:
     - Posture and positioning
     - Speech therapy: oral awareness and oral motor skills training
     - Behavioural therapy
     - Pharmacotherapy: anticholinergic, antihistamines, antireflux, botulinum toxin
   - Surgical:
     - Submandibular duct rerouting, submandibular duct excision, parotid duct ligation, submandibular duct ligation and transtympanic neuronectomy.

CASE 82

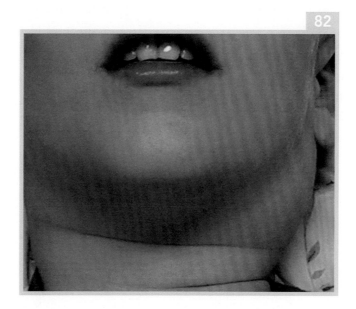

A 5-year-old boy presents with a high fever for 5 days, irritability, conjunctival injection, erythema of his hands, feet and tongue and an enlarged neck node.

i.   What is the diagnosis?

ii. What is the underlying etiology?

iii. What is the most concerning complication?

iv. How is this treated?

Answers 82

i. Kawasaki disease.

ii. It is an autoimmune disease in which the medium-sized blood vessels throughout the body become inflamed.

iii. Left untreated the mortality may approach 1%. The most concerning complications are cardiac such as coronary artery aneurysm and acute myocardial infarct.

iv. Multidisciplinary input from the paediatric and cardiology team is important. Treatment is typically intravenous immunoglobulin (IVIG). Corticosteroids are used when the disease is resistant to IVIG.

CASE 83

QUESTIONS 83

You are working at the regional paediatric ENT hospital and the following child with craniosynostosis attends your clinic with her parents.

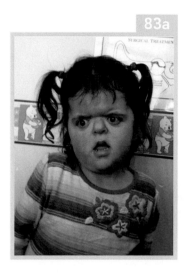

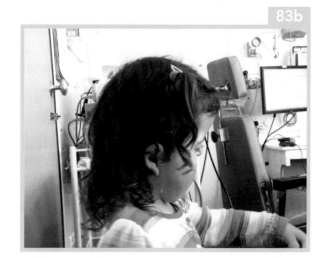

i.   What is craniosynostosis?

ii.   Name some syndromal causes of craniosynostosis and syndrome specific features?

iii. Which sutures can fuse prematurely and what name is given to the cranial shape when that occurs?

iv.   Which other surgical specialties typically are involved in the multidisciplinary care of these children?

i. Craniosynostosis is premature fusion of the sutures of the skull. This prevents normal skull expansion and results in deformity of the skull or, if all sutures fuse prematurely, microcephaly.

ii. Syndromes associated with craniosynostosis include the following:
  - Crouzon syndrome: low-set ears, brachycephaly, exophthalmos, hypertelorism, divergent strabismus, maxillary hypoplasia
  - Apert syndrome: similar to Crouzon syndrome but with syndactyly
  - Muenke syndrome: coronal synostosis, skeletal abnormalities
  - Pfeiffer syndrome: broad, short thumbs/toes

iii. Sutures affected are as follows:
  - Sagittal synostosis 50%: scaphocephaly
  - Coronal synostosis 25%: brachycephaly
  - Anterior plagiocephaly: unilateral suture fusion
  - Metopic synostosis 10%: trigonocephaly
  - Lambdoid synostosis 5%: posterior plagiocephalus
  - Complex (multiple sutures affected, usually syndromic) 10%

iv. Maxillofacial and plastic surgeons.

QUESTIONS 84

A 4-week-old baby presents with inspiratory stridor, failure to thrive and choking episodes. Endoscopic appearance is shown as follows.

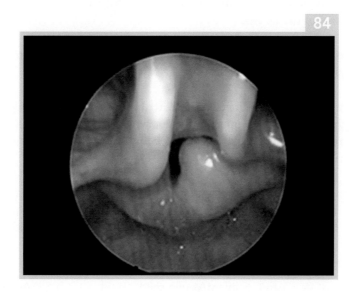

84

i.   What is the diagnosis and what are some of the etiological theories?

ii. What is the classic clinical presentation of this condition?

iii. How does an infant/young child's larynx differ from that of an adult?

iv. How would you classify this condition?

v.   What are the indications for surgical intervention?

i. The condition is laryngomalacia.

There are three postulated theories of etiology:

a. The neuromuscular immaturity theory is the most accepted theory. It suggests that laryngeal hypotonia occurs due to delayed neuromuscular control of the larynx.

b. The theory of anatomical abnormality attributes the cause to abnormal laryngeal shape and structure.

c. The cartilage immaturity theory attributes the cause to delayed maturation of the cartilaginous support of the larynx. This theory has been refuted by recent studies that showed normal histology of fibroelastic arytenoid cartilage in affected patients.

ii. The hallmark symptom is inspiratory stridor developing within a few weeks of birth that increases over several months. It is worse in a supine position with crying or feeding. There may be associated feeding difficulties with choking, coughing and regurgitation.

iii.

	Infant/young child	Adult
Position (vertically)	Higher; C1–C4	Lower; C4–C6/C7
Narrowest portion	Cricoid cartilage	Vocal cords
Epiglottis	Longer, more omega shaped and more pliable. Angled more posteriorly	Shorter, wider and more vertically positioned
Vocal folds	Anteroinferior incline Vocal process of arytenoid cartilage occupies ½ of cord	Lie more horizontally Vocal process of arytenoid cartilage occupies ¼ of cord
Cartilage	More pliable	Stiffer

iv. There are many classification systems, but no universal system.

There are four main categories:
- Posterior collapse: the redundant arytenoid mucosa or corniculate cartilages prolapses into the airway
- Lateral collapse: aryepiglottic folds and cuneiform or corniculate cartilages prolapse
- Anterior collapse: obstruction from retroflexed epiglottis
- Combined: two or more of the above patterns coexist

v.   Laryngomalacia is a self-limiting condition in 85%–90% of patients. Absolute indications for surgery include: cor pulmonale/pulmonary hypertension, pectus excavatum, hypoxia/hypercapnia, life-threatening airway obstruction, respiratory compromise and failure to thrive.

Relative indications include: weight loss with feeding difficulty, aspiration and sleep disordered breathing.

QUESTIONS 85

A 7-year-old child presents with painless swelling on his neck over the last 3 weeks.

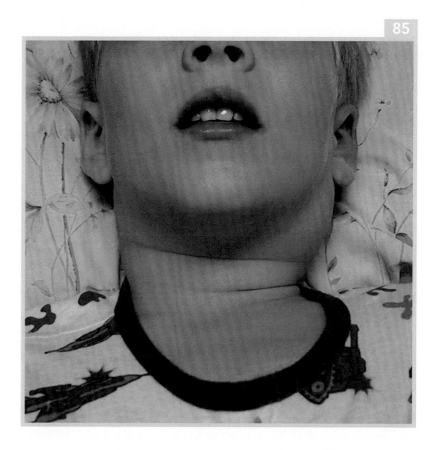

i.   What is the most common benign cause of paediatric lymphadenopathy?

ii.   What are the most common malignancies that present with cervical lymphadenopathy?

iii. What features suggest a malignant process?

iv.   What investigations would you request to investigate persistent cervical lymphadenopathy?

i. A viral upper respiratory tract infection causing reactive lymphadenopathy, for example, rhinovirus, adenovirus, parainfluenza virus, respiratory syncytial virus.

ii. <6 years of age: most commonly neuroblastoma and leukaemia followed by rhabdomyosarcoma and non-Hodgkin's lymphoma.

>6 years of age: Hodgkin's lymphoma is the most common tumour followed by non-Hodgkin's lymphoma and rhabdomyosarcoma.

iii. Lymph node features
   • Position: supraclavicular lymphadenopathy (>50% are malignant)
   • Size: >3 cm or increasing over 2 weeks
   • Persistence despite antibiotics
   • Fixed to skin and deep tissues
   • Not returning to baseline size after 8–12 weeks
 • Generalised lymphadenopathy
 • Hepatosplenomegaly
 • Concurrent symptoms of a systemic disease, for example, malaise, weight loss

iv. A thorough history and examination is essential. Investigations are then tailored to the patient and include the following:
 • Bloods:
   • Full blood count (FBC) (leucocytosis with a bacterial infection, atypical lymphocytes with infectious mononucleosis and leukaemia may show blast cells or pancytopenia).
   • Purified protein derivative (PPD for tuberculosis).
   • Specific serology for Epstein–Barr virus, *Bartonella henselae*, cytomegalovirus, toxoplasmosis.
 • Imaging:
   • Ultrasound scan (USS) is indicated as the initial imaging modality of the neck as it avoids radiation.
   • Chest x-ray (CXR) may show mediastinal lymphadenopathy.
   • Computed tomography (CT) and magnetic resonance imaging (MRI) are helpful with deeper masses.
 • Fine-needle aspiration (FNA):
   It is only useful when it yields a positive result. Performing an FNA in a child who is awake is challenging and the test can be non-diagnostic.
 • Biopsy under general anaesthetic:
   This is the gold standard for a tissue diagnosis and should be performed when the FNA is inconclusive or negative and there is a high suspicion of malignancy.

You are planning a teaching session on paediatric airway management for junior members of the ENT team.

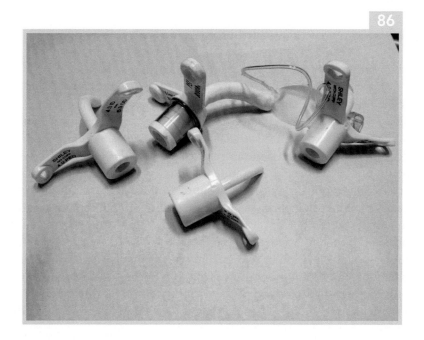

i.   What are shown in the picture?

ii. What are the indications for this procedure?

iii. Describe how this procedure is performed?

iv. What are the complications for this procedure?

i. A selection of paediatric tracheostomy tubes.

ii. There are three main reasons tracheostomy is performed in children:

Prolonged artificial ventilation (e.g. respiratory distress syndrome, neuromuscular disease)

Upper airway obstruction (including congenital and acquired)

Need for pulmonary toilet (e.g. underlying neurological disease)

iii. After the patient is prepared and draped, either a vertical or horizontal skin incision is made just below the level of the cricoid cartilage. The subcutaneous fat is removed. The midline avascular muscular raphe is bluntly divided and dissection is continued until the anterior tracheal wall is identified. The isthmus of the thyroid gland may be encountered and may need to be divided or retracted. Silk or polypropylene 'stay' sutures are placed through the tracheal cartilages on either side of the planned vertical incision in the trachea. These sutures are taped to the chest wall and aid tracheostomy tube change or replacement if there is accidental decannulation. The trachea is typically entered through a vertical incision of two tracheal rings (usually the second and third, or third and fourth). Maturation sutures from the tracheal incision to the vertically incised skin may be performed. The endotracheal tube is slowly retracted under direct visualisation and the tracheostomy tube is inserted and connected to the ventilatory circuit. The tube is then secured.

iv. Complications include the following:

Intra-operative:

Damage to surrounding structures, for example, anterior larynx, anterior or posterior tracheal wall and vessels causing haemorrhage

Post-operative:

Accidental decannulation, pneumomediastinum, pneumothorax, subcutaneous emphysema, haemorrhage, wound infection, skin breakdown, tube plugging, stomal granulation

Post-decannulation:

Tracheocutaneous fistula, tracheomalacia at tracheostomy site, tracheal stenosis.

QUESTIONS 87

This is a photograph of the larynx of a 4-month-old child with stridor.

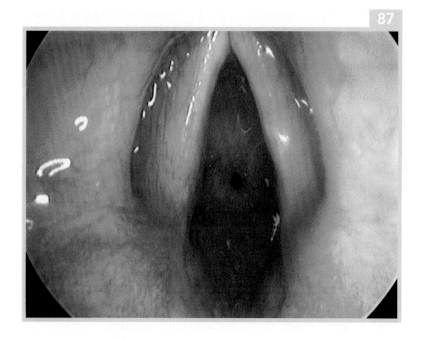

i.   What does the image show?

ii.   What are the causes of this condition?

iii. How is it diagnosed and what findings should be assessed?

iv.   Name and outline any staging systems used to classify this condition?

v.   What are the surgical treatment options?

Answers 87

i. There is a subglottic stenosis with only a pinhole airway remaining. The rest of the larynx looks normal.

ii. Subglottic stenosis can be congenital or acquired.

The common cause of acquired subglottic stenosis is secondary to intubation. It occurs in approximately 1%–2% of intubated children.

Other acquired causes include the following:
- Laryngeal trauma: blunt, penetrating or inhalation (thermal or caustic)
- Iatrogenic: airway surgery
- Autoimmune conditions
- Infection
- Gastroesophageal reflux
- Inflammatory conditions such as systemic lupus erythematosus (SLE) and sarcoidosis

iii. The gold standard for diagnosis of any laryngotracheal abnormality is direct laryngoscopy and tracheobronchoscopy under general anaesthesia.

The important things to document during endoscopy are as follows:
- Circumferential size of the stenotic segment that may be assessed by documenting the outer diameter of the largest bronchoscope or endotracheal tube that can be passed through the stenotic segment.
- Location/sub-sites (glottis, subglottis, trachea) and length of the stenosis.
- Other separate sites of stenosis.
- Other airway anomalies in infants, for example, clefts, webs, cricoarytenoid joint fixation, neoplasms.
- Reflux changes.
- Oedema developing in the stenotic segment after removing the sizing endotracheal tube or bronchoscope because this may result in the need for a tracheostomy.

iv. There are two classification systems that can be used:

Myer–Connor–Cotton classification:

This describes the degree of stenosis based on the relative percentage reduction in cross-sectional area compared to the normal trachea.
- 0%–50%
- 51%–70%
- 71%–99%
- No detectable lumen

McCaffrey system:

Laryngotracheal stenosis is staged based on the sub-sites involved and the length of the stenosis.
- Confined to the subglottis or trachea, <1 cm long
- Confined to the subglottis, >1 cm long
- Subglottic/tracheal lesions not involving the glottis
- Involves the glottis

v.   Surgical treatment can be endoscopic or open surgery.

Endoscopic treatment includes dilatation or endoscopic excision of the stenosis and may be performed with cold steel or a CO_2 laser.

Open procedures can be classified as either expansion, resection or a tracheostomy.

Expansion can be performed as a single stage or with stent placement. They range from an anterior and/or posterior cricoid split (laryngotracheoplasty) to a four-quadrant division of the cricoid cartilage. Cartilage graft may be inserted to increase expansion (laryngotracheal reconstruction).

Resection of the affected segment is called cricotracheal resection and may be performed in conjunction with an expansion procedure.

QUESTIONS 88

A child presents to the emergency department with pyrexial illness and drooling too. A lateral soft-tissue x-ray has been taken.

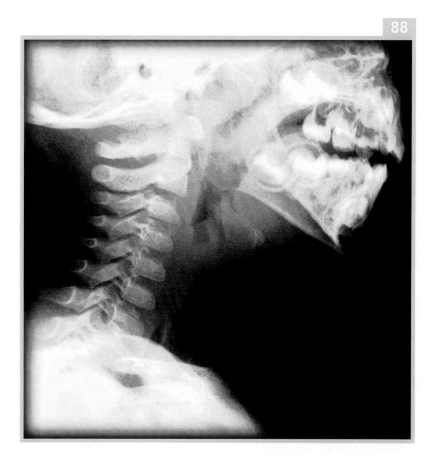

i.   What does this show?

ii.   What are the typical presenting features?

iii. What is the emergency management of this condition?

i.   This shows the 'thumb print' sign suggesting the diagnosis of epiglottitis – it is caused by a thickened free edge of the epiglottis, which causes it to appear more radiopaque than normal, resembling the distal thumb. In reality, this patient should not have been sent for this investigation, as the airway is unstable.

ii.   The typical patient is a child aged 2 to 4 years with sore throat, stridor, muffled voice, dysphagia leading to drooling, pyrexia with sepsis.

iii. Acute epiglottitis is a potentially life-threatening disease due to upper airway soft-tissue obstruction and sepsis. Patients with typical symptoms should be identified early. The child should be kept with his or her parents and distress should be minimised. Oxygen and adrenaline nebulisers should be held nearby but not by a tight fitting mask. A consultant paediatric anaesthetist, a paediatrician and a senior ENT surgeon should all be present. The child should be transferred urgently to the operating room and after slow gaseous anaesthetic induction with spontaneous breathing a careful laryngoscopy should be carried out. The child should be intubated with an endotracheal tube. The child should then be managed in the paediatric intensive care unit with appropriate intravenous (IV) antibiotics and repeat laryngoscopy when signs of sepsis and laryngeal swelling are subsiding.

CASE 89

QUESTIONS 89

A 3-year-old child presents to your clinic with a history of loud snoring and witnessed episodes of apnoea. Clinical examination reveals the following.

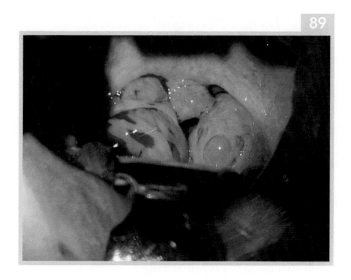

i. What does the image show?

ii. Do you know any grading systems for tonsillar size?

iii. What are signs and symptoms of paediatric obstructive sleep apnoea (OSA)?

iv. What potential complications can occur?

v. What is the usual definitive treatment for paediatric OSA?

vi. In more severe cases what other treatment options are there?

vii. What syndromes are associated with OSA?

i.   Large obstructing tonsils touching in the midline.

ii.   Mallampati grading:

Tonsil 0: tonsil fits within tonsillar fossa

Tonsil 1: tonsils are less than 25% of space between pillars

Tonsil 2: tonsils are less than 50% of space between pillars

Tonsil 3: tonsils are less than 75% of space between pillars

Tonsil 4: tonsils are more than 75% of space between pillars

Friedman grading (tongue in neutral position):

Tonsil 0: a previous tonsillectomy has been performed

Tonsil 1: tonsils hidden between the tonsillar pillars

Tonsil 2: tonsils extend to the tonsillar pillars

Tonsil 3: tonsils extend beyond the pillars but not to the midline

Tonsil 4: tonsils extend to the midline

iii.   Snoring with restless sleep and unusual 'posturing' sleeping position. Reduced breathing for one or two breaths followed by gasping for air often with minor arousal from sleep.

Mouth breathing at night and often when awake also.

iv.   Poor quality sleep may lead to any of the following: daytime sleepiness, poor concentration, enuresis, decreased intellectual ability and behavioural difficulties.

Failure to thrive.

Prolonged hypoxaemia and hypercarbia leads to pulmonary hypertension and right heart failure.

v.   Adenotonsillectomy.

vi.   Nasal treatment if nasal obstruction (i.e. rhinitis, nasal polyps)

Sleeping in the prone position may help. If there is nasal obstruction (eg. chronic rhinosinusitis) then treatment of the underlying nasal pathology may also help. Other interventions that may be considered include the following:

- Continuous positive airway pressure (CPAP)
- Prone positioning
- Nasopharyngeal airway
- Maxillomandibular surgery
- Tongue base surgery
- Tracheostomy

vii. The calibre of the upper airway may be compromised in the following conditions which may result in OSA:

- Down syndrome
- Pierre–Robin
- Treacher–Collins
- Achondroplasia
- Cerebral palsy
- Mucopolysaccharidosis
- Craniofacial syndromes
- Many neuromuscular disorders.

CASE 90

A 6-year-old boy presents to the emergency department with swelling around the right eye.

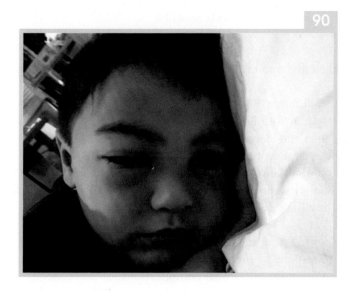

This has been present for 24 hours and is associated with a high temperature and tachycardia. He has had cold over the preceding week.

i.   What is your differential diagnosis?

ii.   How would you manage this patient initially?

iii. When would you request imaging?

iv.   Do you know how to classify this condition?

i.   This is a clinical picture showing pre-septal cellulitis of the right eye. The differential diagnosis would include the following:
- Inflammation: eczema, allergic conjunctivitis, insect bite. Local allergic reaction
- Infection: secondary infection to the above plus localised skin infections, lid infections, dacrocyctitis, acute sinusitis
- Trauma

ii.
- Admit the child and initiate antibiotic therapy according to local hospital policy.
- Topical nasal steroids and decongestants.
- Send bloods for: full blood count (FBC), C-reactive protein (CRP), blood culture, urea and electrolytes (U&E) test.
- Swab the eye for culture and sensitivity.
- Formal ophthalmology review if possible (particularly colour vision and acuity). Colour vision is checked using Ishihara charts. Check for a relative afferent pupillary defect.

iii.   Indications for CT scan include the following:
- Failure to respond to medical therapy over a 24-hour period
- Signs and symptoms of orbital complications:
  - Proptosis, chemosis, ophthalmoplegia, exophthalmos, decreased visual acuity, loss of red/green colour vision and afferent pupillary reflex (latter three are late signs with imminent threat to vision due to raised orbital pressure and compromised blood flow to the optic nerve)
- Signs and symptoms of intracranial complications:
  - Photophobia, meningism, confusion, altered Glasgow Coma Scale, seizures, focal neurological signs
- Inability to examine the eye and suspicion of post-septal cellulitis
- An MRI scan is indicated if there are symptoms or signs of cerebritis, brain abscess or cavernous sinus thrombosis (bilateral proptosis, chemosis, photophobia, temperature, ophthalmoplegia, loss of vision, hypothesia in the distribution of the ophthalmic and maxillary divisions of the trigeminal nerve.

iv.   The most common classification for orbital cellulitis is Chandler's classification:
- Group I: pre-septal cellulitis
- Group II: orbital cellulitis
- Group III: subperiosteal abscess
- Group IV: orbital abscess
- Group V: cavernous sinus thrombosis

CASE 91

QUESTIONS 91

A 3-year-old child is referred to clinic because of a blocked nose; the general practitioner is querying if the adenoids are enlarged and need removing.

On examination, this is what you find.

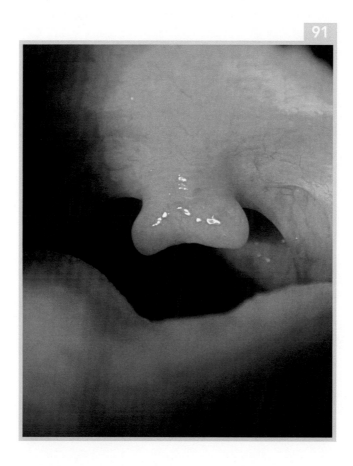

i.   What does the picture show?

ii.   What is the embryological origin for this?

iii.   What specific complication could result if an adenoidectomy is performed in this child?

i.   A bifid uvula.

ii.   A bifid uvula results from incomplete fusion of the palatine shelves. It may be associated with a submucous cleft (visible or occult) and cleft palate.

iii.   Velopharygeal insufficiency. This is characterised by hypernasal speech, nasal emission and turbulence and occasionally nasal regurgitation of fluids.

CASE 92

QUESTIONS 92

A 15-year-old girl complains of a sore throat and is unable to eat or drink. She is pyrexial at 39°C and has bilateral tender cervical lymphadenopathy.

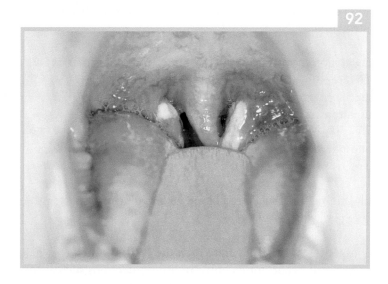

i.   What is the likely diagnosis?

ii. What is the cause of this condition?

iii. How would you test for it?

i. There is bilateral exudate on both tonsils. In view of the high temperature and significant lymphadenopathy, the diagnosis is likely to be glandular fever rather than acute tonsillitis.

ii. Epstein–Barr virus (EBV): the virus is approximately 120–180 nm in diameter and is composed of a double helix of DNA wrapped in a protein capsid.

iii. A full blood count may show raised white cell count with a lymphocytosis rather than neutrophilia.

Infectious mononucleosis causes heterophile antibodies to form in the patient's serum. Heterophile antibodies means that antibodies against an antigen produced in one species reacts against antigens from another species. This phenomenon can be used to diagnose glandular fever. Examples include:

The Monospot test: horse red blood cells agglutinate on exposure to heterophile antibodies.

The Paul–Bunnell test: sheep red blood cells agglutinate in the presence of heterophile antibodies.

The Monospot test is more accurate than the Paul–Bunnell test. False positives can, however, still occur, for example in other infections such as toxoplasmosis, rubella, human immunodeficiency virus (HIV), Burkitt lymphoma and connective tissue disease, such as rheumatoid arthritis. False negatives can also occur if performed too early in the course of the disease or in very young children.

A more accurate test is to look for EBV-specific antibodies. The most useful EBV-specific antibodies are the viral capsid antigens (VCAs) and the EBV nuclear antigen (EBNA) and more recently real-time polymerase chain reaction (PCR) analysis can be used.

QUESTIONS 93

This is a photograph of the post-nasal space in a baby who was born with breathing difficulties. Paediatricians are unable to pass a nasogastric tube through either nostril.

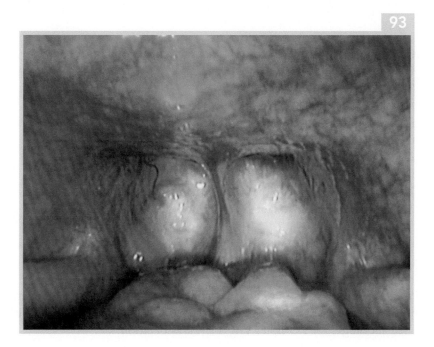

i.   What is the diagnosis and what statistics do you know about the condition?

ii.   What syndrome is it associated with and what other pathologies can occur in that syndrome?

iii.   What is the difference between a sequence, an association and a syndrome?

iv.   How would you manage this child?

i. Bilateral choanal atresia

This condition affects 1 in 8000 births and is more common in girls than boys (2:1). It is more often unilateral rather than bilateral (2:1) and in unilateral cases it is more common on the right. Seventy percent are a combination of soft tissue and bone. Thirty percent are purely bony. Purely membranous atresia is very rare.

ii. The condition is associated with CHARGE syndrome. This consists of:
- Coloboma of the eye
- Heart defects
- Atresia of the nasal choanae
- Retardation of growth/development
- Genital/urological abnormalities
- Ear abnormalities/deafness
- 50% of CHARGE patients have some sort of choanal atresia
- 75% of bilateral choanal atresia patients have other CHARGE defects
- 36% of unilateral choanal atresia patients have other CHARGE defects

iii. A sequence is a condition where one abnormality occurs, which causes a cascade of further abnormalities, for example, Pierre–Robin.

An association is a non-random pattern of abnormalities that occur together more commonly than expected but are developmental, unrelated and with no defined aetiology, for example, VACTERL association.

A syndrome has multiple unrelated abnormalities with a proven cause such as genetic link, for example, Down syndrome (Trisomy 21).

CHARGE syndrome used to be categorised as an association but in 2004 a genetic cause was proven (*CHD7* gene on Chromosome 8 [67% of cases]), which means that it is now deemed a CHARGE syndrome.

iv. An oropharyngeal airway should be inserted immediately after birth to maintain the airway as neonates are obligate nasal breathers. This will need to be followed by staged endoscopic and/or transpalatal surgery to recanalise the choanae.

This is a photograph of a 5-year-old boy with a history of snoring.

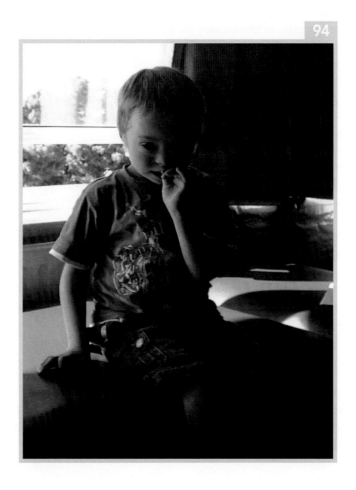

i. What is the diagnosis?

ii. How can this be inherited?

iii. What are the ENT manifestations seen in this condition?

iv. What general manifestations might you expect this child to have?

i. Trisomy 21 (also known as Down syndrome).

ii. Trisomy 21 is not usually an inherited condition. The trisomy occurs as a random event and results from a meiotic non-dysjunction event. This results in the the production of an extra copy of chromosome 21. In around 5% of cases it may inherited and in these cases the genetic defect is a translocation between chromosome 14 and chromosome 21. Trisomy 21 may in some cases also show mosaicism. If the non-dysjunction occurs during early cell division of the embryo, ie. is not present at fertilisation, then only some of the cells in the body carry the genetic defect. The phenotype is usually milder.

iii. ENT manifestations include:

Ears: narrow external auditory canal (EAC), otitis media with effusion (OME), ossicular chain abnormalities, inner ear abnormalities with sensorineural deafness, small pinna

Nose: chronic rhinitis, sinusitis (abnormalities of serum immunoglobulins and ciliary dyskinesia), poor Eustachian tube function

Throat: large tonsils and adenoids, short posterior nasal spine, macroglossia, airway obstruction, obstructive sleep apnoea, subglottic stenosis, atlanto-axial instability

iv. General manifestations include:

Microgenia (round face), epicanthal folds, Brushfield spots (white spots on iris), upslanting palpebral fissures, shorter limbs, a single transverse palmar crease, poor muscle tone, learning disabilities (IQ variable 20–85), joint laxity, atlanto-axial instability, cardiac abnormalities (atrioventricular septal defects 40%).

CASE 95

A 5-year-old boy presents to the accident and emergency department at 10 PM following a choking episode that lasted a few minutes. It was unwitnessed but was heard by his grandmother who was in the next room. Clinically he appears well but his grandmother says he has a 'funny' noise when he breathes in deeply. Oxygen saturations are 99% on room air and he is speaking normally.

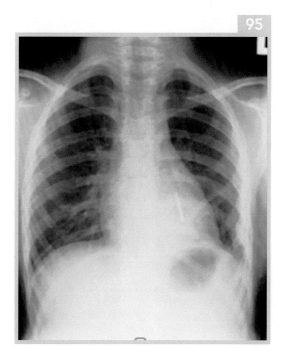

i.   What does the chest x-ray show?

ii. How would you manage this?

i.   There is a foreign body in the left bronchus.

ii.   The object needs removal via a bronchoscopy. The question is when and where
      it should be performed. If he is clinically stable, removal could wait until the
      next morning and be performed on an ENT list where the operating room
      team/anaesthetist will be familiar with the equipment required to carry out the
      procedure. If he is in a district general hospital without a paediatric anaesthetist,
      it could be argued that he should be transferred to a paediatric ENT centre
      and the procedure done on the following day. If there is significant airway
      compromise the child should be transferred urgently to a paediatric ENT centre
      and the procedure should be carried out on arrival.

CASE 96

QUESTIONS 96

A 3-month-old child presents with stridor. He was born at term with no specific prenatal, perinatal or postnatal problems. This is the appearance at direct laryngotracheobronchoscopy (DLTB).

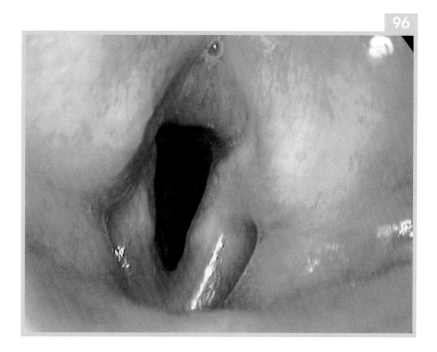

i.   What is the diagnosis and what non-airway manifestations are there for this condition?

ii. What is the typical time course of presentation and natural history?

iii. What medical treatment is now used first line in most cases?

iv. What parameters must be investigated or monitored initially?

i.   The diagnosis is subglottic haemangioma.

        50% of subglottic haemangiomas have associated cutaneous haemangiomas.

        5% of cutaneous haemangiomas have associated subglottic haemangiomas.

ii.   They usually increase in size and cause symptoms (stridor) around 6 weeks after
        birth. They increase in size up to 18 months old then plateau in size. Gradual
        spontaneous involution occurs after that so that half resolve by age 5 and all by
        age 10.

iii.   Propanolol. The efficacy in this condition was an incidental finding and its
        mechanism of action is unknown.

iv.   The parameters include blood pressure, performing an echocardiogram, an
        ultrasound to check the renal arteries and kidneys, blood glucose, weight (to
        judge dose and increase dose as weight increases with age). This condition is
        often managed in conjunction with the paediatric team.

CASE 97

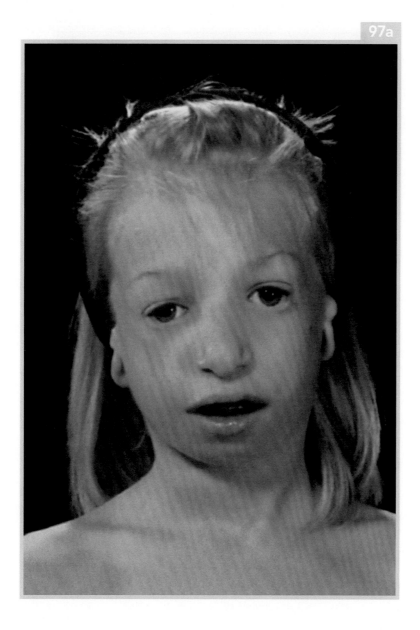

QUESTIONS 97

This 6-year-old girl attends your outpatient clinic for the first time having just moved recently to the local area.

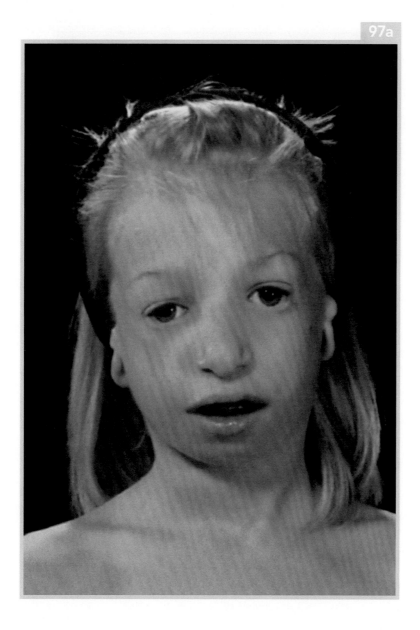

97a

i.   What is the diagnosis? What is the inheritance pattern and incidence?

ii.   What are the general features seen in this condition?

iii. What ENT problems might you expect this child to have?

The same child has this appearance of her pinna.

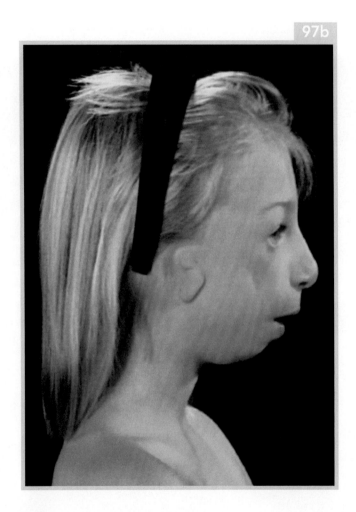

iv.   What does it show?

v.   Is there a classification system for this?

vi.   What are the treatment options?

Answers 97

i. Treacher–Collins syndrome, an autosomal dominant condition with the mutation occurring in the TCOF1 gene. It has a prevalence of 1 in 50,000.

ii.
- Hypoplasia of the facial bones including mandible
- Down slanting palpebral fissures
- Vision loss with strabismus
- Cleft palate
- Normal intelligence
- Dental anomalies

iii.
- Airway obstruction (micrognathia and cleft palate)
- Microtia + canal atresia
- Conductive deafness due to canal atresia and ossicular malformation
- Auricular pits, fistulas and tags

iv. Microtia and canal atresia

v. Alteman's classification is the most widely used. It categorises atresia into 3 types:

Type 1: Mild. A meatus and tympanic membrane exist but are often small. The ossicular chain is usually fixed and the stapes is abnormal.

Type 2: Moderate. The pinna is severely deformed and the ear canal is absent. There is significant anomaly of the ossicular chain.

Type 3: Severe. The pinna is rudimentary or absent and the ear canal is absent. The mastoid is under-pneumatised.

vi. Treatment has multiple considerations:

Hearing: bone-conducting or bone-anchored hearing aids (BAHAs) work well as the hearing loss is often mostly conductive. (The surgical position of the BAHA should be sufficiently posterior to allow for future reconstructive surgical options.)

Pinna cosmesis: this should be considered when the child is old enough to be part of the discussion.

- Prosthetic ear fitting: this provides a good aesthetic ear but it gets clipped on and off and needs changing with age and suntan and so on. It requires surgical titanium implants for placement.
- Surgical ear reconstruction: this is usually performed in three or four surgical stages. Autologous rib graft is harvested and carved to form the skeleton of the pinna. It is then inserted subcutaneously. Results show a good pseudo-natural ear that grows with the patient and tans in sunshine and so on. If they have a BAHA, then this must be posteriorly placed to allow a subcutaneous pocket to be developed.

Canal atresia: surgical canal reconstruction often re-stenoses. A preoperative computed tomography (CT) scan is needed to assess the dura, facial nerve course and middle ear anatomy. Surgical success is based on restoration of useful hearing, long-term stability of hearing and maintenance of a patent, skin-lined ear canal. The Jahrsdoerfer 10-point grading system is used to determine surgical candidacy and is based on key features from the CT scan and the appearance of the external ear. This system is also used to indirectly estimate the likelihood of success if surgical correction is performed. With the highly successful nature of BAHA, conservative treatment is often chosen to avoid the risks associated with canal atresia reconstruction.

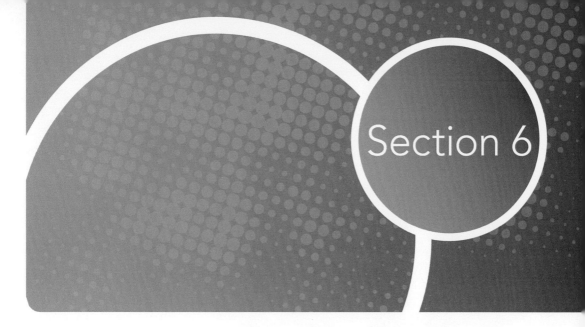

Section 6

MISCELLANEOUS

QUESTIONS 98

A 43-year-old woman has a granuloma on her left buccal mucosa secondary to an ill-fitting denture. You are going to be removing it under local anaesthetic.

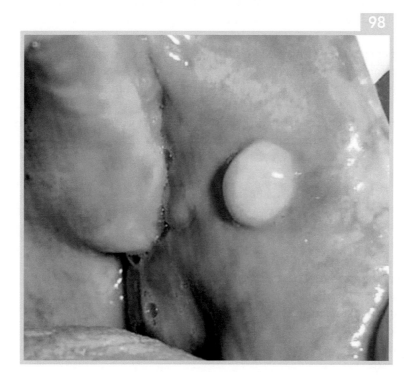

i.   What is the maximum dose of the following local anaesthetics?
  • Lignocaine
  • Lignocaine with adrenaline
  • Bupivacaine
  • Bupivacaine with adrenaline

ii.   What is EMLA and Ametop?

iii. What are the symptoms of local anaesthetic toxicity?

iv.   What monitoring is required during local anaesthetic procedures?

i. Lignocaine 300 mg: 4–5 mg/kg
    Lignocaine with adrenaline 500 mg: 7 mg/kg
    Bupivacaine 175 mg: 2.5 mg/kg
    Bupivacaine with adrenaline 225 mg: 3 mg/kg

ii. EMLA stands for Eutectic Mixture of Local Anaesthetics. It is a combination of 2.5% lidocaine and 2.5% prilocaine. Ametop is 4% tetracaine.

iii. Toxic effects can be divided into local and general types. Local toxicity manifests as:
    • Prolonged anaesthesia
    • Prolonged parasthesia (tingling, feeling of 'pins and needles')

    General toxic effects occur if there is systemic absorption that effects the central nervous system or the cardiovascular system and include:

    Central nervous system effects

    The effects may be excitatory or depressant depending on the concentration of the anaesthetic. Side effects include:
    • Tinnitus
    • Metallic taste in mouth
    • Tingling or numbness in the mouth
    • Motor twitching
    • Grand mal seizures
    • Coma
    • Respiratory arrest
    • Death

    Cardiovascular effects

    • Hypotension
    • Atrioventricular conduction delay
    • Arrythmias
    • Cardiac collapse

iv. Minimum monitoring required is pulse oximetry, non-invasive blood pressure monitor and electrocardiograph.

A patient is about to undergo a local anaesthetic procedure and a member of the theatre team is attaching monitoring to the patient.

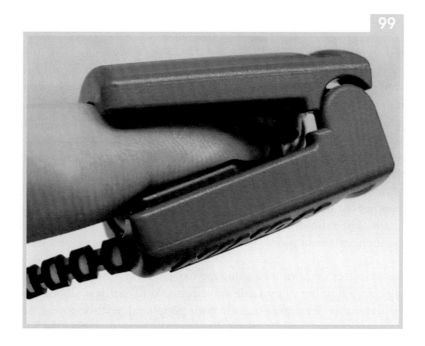

i.   What is this machine and what does it measure?

ii.   Can you explain the principle of how this machine works?

iii. When may its reading not be reliable?

i. A pulse oximeter – it measures oxygen saturation.

ii. Pulse oximeters provide a measurement of oxygen saturation of haemoglobin within the circulation. Four molecules of oxygen combine with one molecule of haemoglobin to form oxyhaemoglobin. The oximeter is able to measure and thus differentiate the absorption of specific wavelengths of light in oxygenated haemoglobin, as compared with that of reduced deoxyhaemoglobin.

Arterial oxygenated blood is bright red due to the oxyhaemoglobin it contains, causing it to absorb light of certain wavelengths. The oximeter probe has two light-emitting diodes (LEDs), one red and one infrared, located on one side of the probe. The probe is placed on a suitable part of the body – usually a fingertip or ear lobe – and the LEDs transmit the two wavelengths through pulsating arterial blood to a photodetector on the other side of the probe. Infrared light is absorbed preferentially by the oxyhaemoglobin; red light by the reduced deoxyhaemoglobin. Pulsatile arterial blood during systole causes an influx of oxyhaemoglobin to the tissue, absorbing more infrared light; meaning less red light reaches the photodetector. The opposite occurs if the oxygen content of the blood falls. The ratio of absorbed infrared to red light is processed into a digital display of oxygen saturation.

iii. A pulse oximeter determines a value for oxygen saturation based on an average reading over a number of pulsatile waveforms. Where this is altered, the value may be unreliable. Examples include poor peripheral perfusion, such as in hypovolaemic or cardiogenic shock. Tachycardia may also affect the accuracy of the oximeter.

From the oxygen–haemaglobin dissociation curve, a small decrease in partial pressure of oxygen at around 92% oxygen saturation results in a rapid dissociation of oxygen from haemoglobin and an exponential fall in saturation. Therefore, between 70% and 90% saturations, the oximeter reading may be inaccurate. This is of significance in conditions such as cyanotic congenital cardiac disease.

Pulse oximeters can give a falsely high reading if carbon monoxide is present. Carbon monoxide binds to haemoglobin approximately 250 times more strongly than oxygen and, once in place, prevents the binding of oxygen. It also turns haemoglobin bright red. The pulse oximeter is unable to distinguish between haemoglobin molecules saturated in oxygen and those carrying carbon monoxide.

Pulse oximeters do not offer information about haemoglobin concentration, cardiac output, efficiency of oxygen delivery to the tissues, oxygen consumption, sufficiency of oxygenation or adequacy of ventilation.

CASE 100

A 7-year-old boy is first on your operating list for grommet insertion. You are checking the microscope and setting your inter-pupillary distance. This piece of equipment is just behind the microscope.

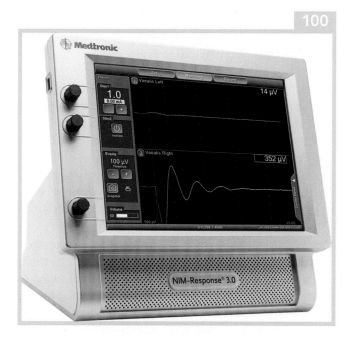

i. What is this piece of equipment and give examples of surgery where it can be useful?

ii. What are the physiological principles of using this machine?

i. This is a nerve monitor. It is used to monitor nerves in the head and neck region during surgery that may put the relevent nerve at risk. Examples of situations where this type of nerve monitoring may be useful are:

Thyroid surgery (to monitor the recurrent laryngeal nerves using a special endotracheal tube)

Parotid surgery (to monitor the facial nerve)

Mastoid surgery (to monitor the facial nerve)

ii. Continuous neurophysiological monitoring evaluates the electromyographic activity. There are two types of potential responses: non-repetitive and repetitive.

Non-repetitive responses are produced by direct mechanical or electrical stimulation of the facial nerve. Electrical stimulation is usually with a monopolar probe where the current flows from the stimulation probe in all directions (vs. a bipolar probe where the current flows only between the tips). Although bipolar probes are more precise as less current is shunted away, it will only stimulate the nerve if the nerve lies directly between the two tips. Monopolar probes are insulated flush to the tip to minimise current shunting; blood or irrigation fluid have a low impedance so should be removed prior to stimulation again to prevent current shunting. The amplitude of the stimulus needed depends upon the site of stimulation. For example, during facial nerve monitoring in acoustic neuroma surgery, the stimulus at the brainstem is usually 0.05 mA; however, in mastoid surgery, a stimulus of 1 mA may be used to stimulate the vertical segment of the facial nerve in its bony canal.

Repetitive responses (also known as 'training') occur as a result of repetitive depolarisations. Such responses may indicate increased irritability as a result of injury. They cannot be used to locate the nerve but can warn the operating surgeon that injury has occurred or is imminent.

CASE 101

You are teaching medical students how to suture an ear laceration. They ask you about the different types of needles and suture materials.

i.   Label the following parts of a needle.

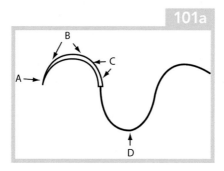

101a

ii.   How can sutures be classified?

iii.   What is the difference between a cutting, reverse cutting and tapered needle?

Answers 101

i.

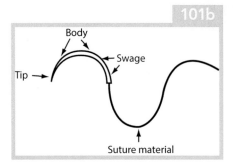

101b

Body

Swage

Tip

Suture material

ii.   Sutures can be classified as natural or synthetic, absorbable or non–absorbable and monofilament or multifilament.

Natural sutures can be made of animal collagen (e.g. mammal intestines) or from synthetic collagen (polymers). They cause inflammatory reactions because of suture antigenicity and subsequent tissue reaction.

Synthetic suture features are listed in the following table.

	Monofilament	Braided	Comment
Number of strands	Single	Multiple	–
Resistance through tissue	Less	More	–
Risk of infection	Less	More	Multifilament sutures have increased capillarity (fluid absorption) therefore may introduce pathogens
Handling	Crushing/crimping may weaken suture	More robust	Multifilament sutures have a higher coefficient of friction therefore may be coated to improve passage through tissue
Tensile strength	Less	More	–

Suture absorption occurs by enzymatic degradation in natural materials and by hydrolysis in synthetic materials. Hydrolysis causes less tissue reaction than enzymatic degradation.

The ideal suture has the following characteristics: sterile, minimal tissue reaction, easy to handle, knots securely, high tensile strength, favorable absorption profile and is resistant to infection.

iii. Conventional cutting needles have three cutting edges (triangular cross section that changes to a flattened body). The third cutting edge is on the inner, concave curvature (surface-seeking). It is ideal for skin suturing.

In reverse-cutting needles, the third cutting edge is on the outer convex curvature of the needle (depth-seeking). These needles are stronger than conventional cutting needles and have a reduced risk of cutting out tissue; therefore causing minimal trauma. The needles are designed for tissue that is tough to penetrate, for example, skin, tendon sheaths, oral mucosa.

Taper-point (round) needles penetrate and pass through tissues by stretching without cutting. A sharp tip at the point flattens to an oval/rectangular shape. The taper-point needle is used for easily penetrated tissues (e.g. subcutaneous layers, dura, peritoneum, abdominal viscera) and minimises the potential tearing of fascia.

QUESTIONS 102

The first patient on your theatre list is for an excision of a left vocal cord tumour (staged T1 N0 M0).

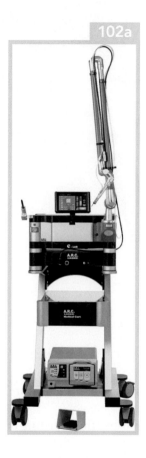

102a

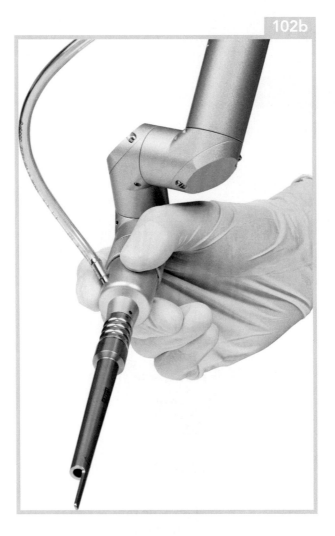

i.   What piece of equipment is shown in the picture?

ii.   What are the advantages in using this machine in head and neck surgery?

iii. What precautions must be taken when using this equipment?

iv.   What would you do in the event of an airway fire?

i.   This is a CO$_2$ laser.

ii.   A CO$_2$ laser has excellent cutting properties. It also causes minimal adjacent tissue damage with very good coagulation properties. At a wavelength of 10,600 nm, it emits a coherent, monochromatic, invisible light with negligible reflection and excellent tissue absorption.

iii. Precautions during laser laryngeal surgery include the presence of a designated laser safety officer; covering the patient's eyes and face with moist compresses; theatre personnel to wear laser safety glasses; doors signed and locked; fume extractor; the use of special endotracheal (ET) tubes (non–inflammable material); ET tube cuff filled with a dye and covered with moist patties; and a bucket of water.

iv.   If an airway fire should occur, the immediate measure is to disconnect the ventilation hose and tracheal tube. Next, the ET tube is removed and saline is sprayed into the airway. Once the fire is extinguished, the patient is immediately re-intubated and a laryngotracheobronchoscopy is performed followed by any necessary critical care measure required.

INDEX

Dacrocystorhinostomy (DCR), 204
Dehiscent carotid artery, 116
Dermatographia, 184
Diffuse involvement of temporal bone, 122
Direct laryngoscopy, 31, 236
'Double ring' sign, 113
Down syndrome, 252, 254
Doxycycline, 212
Draf 2b procedure, 206
Drooling, 222, 240
Dysplasia, 70–71

EBV, *see* Epstein–Barr virus
Ectopic carotid artery, 116
Electrical stimulation, 270
Electrolyte monitoring, 34
Electromyography (EMG) testing, 119
Electronystagmogram (ENG), 99, 127
EMLA (Eutectic Mixture of Local
        Anaesthetics), 266
Endoscopic decompression, 88
Endoscopic dilatation, 52
Endoscopic endonasal approach, 204, 206
Endoscopic sinus surgery, 210, 212
Endoscopic stapling, 52
Endoscopic surgery, 192, 237
Endotracheal (ET) tubes, 277
Epidermoid cysts, 76
Epidermoid tumours, 138
Epiglottitis, 240
Epstein–Barr virus (EBV), 176, 250
Epulis fissuratum, 28
ET tubes, *see* Endotracheal tubes

Facial nerve function, 120, 139
Facial nerve schwannoma, 119, 120
Facial palsy rate, 140
Fascial condensation, 42
Fenestrated tubes, 8
Fibroproliferative disorders, 180
Fibrous dysplasia, 122
Fine-needle aspiration (FNA), 232
Fine needle aspiration cytology (FNAC), 4
Fistula, 90
    testing, 124
Flexible nasendoscopy, 70, 200
Fluorescein lumbar puncture, 200
Fluoride treatment, 113
Fractionated radiotherapy, 140
Free grafts, 200
Frey syndrome, 12, 30, 160
Friedman grading, 242

Frontal sinus, 206
    infection, 167
    median drainage procedures of, 192
Fusobacterium, 42

Gamma Knife machine, 140
Gaze-evoked nystagmus, 101
Genetic testing, 202
Geniculate ganglion, 119, 120
Glomus tumour, 116
Glottis, 32, 237
Grade of roughness, breathiness, asthenia and
        strain (GRBAS), 80
Granulomas, 197
GRBAS, *see* Grade of roughness, breathiness,
        asthenia and strain
'Ground glass' computed tomography,
        122

Haematoma, 146
Haemophilus influenzae, 42
Head thrust test, 99, 103, 104
Hearing, 261
    destructive approaches, 110
    loss, 137
    rehabilitation options, 113
Hemifacial spasm, 160
Hillocks of His, 90
Histamine, 184
Hodgkin's lymphoma, 232
Holger's classification, 94
Horizontal nystagmus, 129
Horner syndrome, 104, 129, 162
Human papillomavirus (HPV), 4, 74, 78
Hydrocephalus, 101
Hyperintense, 110
Hypertrophic scars, 180

Iatrogenic injury, 68
Ideal suture, 273
Infracochlear approaches, 110
Infralabyrinthine approaches, 110
Inosculation, 146
Intracochlear fibrosis, 113
Intracordal, 76
Intranasal endoscopic approaches, 144
Intravenous (IV) antibiotics, 24, 42, 88, 97,
        240
Intravenous immunoglobulin (IVIG),
        224
Ipratropium bromide nasal spray, 148
IVIG, *see* Intravenous immunoglobulin

Jahrsdoerfer 10-point grading system, 262
Jongkee's formula, 101
Juvenile nasopharyngeal angiofibroma (JNA), 186

Kartagener's syndrome, 150
Kawasaki disease, 224

Lacrimal sac, obstruction of, 204
Laryngomalacia, 228, 229
Laryngoscopy, 240
Laryngotracheal abnormality, 236
Laryngotracheal manifestations, 197
Laryngotracheal stenosis, 237
Laryngotracheobronchoscopy, 257, 277
Laser laryngeal surgery, 277
Lateral collapse, 228
LEDs, *see* Light-emitting diodes
Le Fort classification, 170
Le Fort II (pyramidal), 170
Le Fort III (cranial facial dysjunction), 170
Leukotriene antagonists, 212
Ligation, 35, 194
Light-emitting diodes (LEDs), 268
LINAC, *see* Linear accelerator
Linear accelerator (LINAC), 140
5-Lipoxygenase inhibitors, 212
Local anaesthetic, 265, 266
Low maxillary fracture, 170
Ludwig's angina, 23
Lymphadenopathy, 232, 250
Lymphatic malformation, 220
Lymph node metastasis, 39
Lymph nodes, 42, 232
Lynch–Howarth incision, 88

Magnetic resonance imaging (MRI), 46, 144, 206
Mallampati grading, 242
Maxillary fracture, 170
Maxillofacial surgery, 226
McCaffrey system, 237
Meningoencephalocoele, 92
Metastasis, 39
Methotrexate, 198
Microdebrider removal, 78
Middle fossa approach, 92, 110, 139
Midline congenital nasal lesions, 144
Migraine-associated vertigo, 129
Minor iodine–starch test, 12
Mixed hearing loss, 84, 122
MMS, *see* Mohs micrographic surgery

Modified radical neck dissections, 38
Mohs micrographic surgery (MMS), 164
Monopolar probes, 270
Monospot test, 250
MRI, *see* Magnetic resonance imaging
Mucosal hyperplasia, 28
Mucus retention cysts, 76
Muenke syndrome, 226
Myer–Connor–Cotton subglottic/tracheal stenosis, 236
Mylohyoid muscle, 24, 56, 58

Nasal dermoid, 144
Nasal douching, 150, 167, 212
Nasal mucosal oedema, 196
Nasal polyps, 187, 202, 211, 212
Nasal steroids, 202, 246
Nasogastric (NG) tube, 18
Nasolacrimal duct, 204
Natural sutures, 272
Neck swelling, 52
Needle, 271
Neuromuscular immaturity theory, 228
Non-allergic rhinitis, 148
Non-Hodgkin's lymphoma, 232
Non-repetitive responses, 270
Nystagmus, 101, 104, 129

Octreotide, 34
Oesophageal injuries, 49
OK-432, 220
OLP, *see* Oral lichen planus
Opacified mastoid antrum, 97
Oral lichen planus (OLP), 54
Orbital cellulitis, 245
Orlistat, 34
Oropharyngeal manifestations, 197
Osseointegrated bone conduction, 94
Ossification of basal turn, 113
Ossifying haemangiomas, 120
Osteocartilagenous destruction, 196
Osteogenesis imperfecta, 113, 122
Osteoporosis circumcripta, 122
Otogenic abscess, 97
Otological manifestation, 196
Otosclerosis, 107, 113, 122
Oximeter, 268
Oxygen–haemaglobin dissociation curve, 268
Oxyhaemoglobin, 268

Paediatric tracheostomy, 234
Panendoscopy, 4, 48, 49

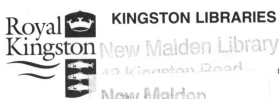

First published in Great Britain in 2001
by HarperCollins Publishers

Westerhill Road

Bishopbriggs

Glasgow G64 2QT

www.**fire**and**water**.com

A catalogue record for this book is available from the
British Library

ISBN 0 00 710235 6

Printed in Great Britain by The Bath Press

CONTENTS

INTRODUCTION

Have you ever been to a job interview? Have you ever been asked to give a presentation to potential clients? To stand up and 'say a few words' about one of your colleagues as she's presented with her leaving present? To speak to a journalist? To speak to your peers at a trade conference?

I expect most people have had to face at least one of these questions and, although you might not have thought about it in this way, they're all forms of public speaking.

Oh – if you said you'd never been asked to do anything like that, watch out! I reckon you're probably next in line.

Your initial instinct might be to say, 'Not on your nelly!' But if your boss tells you your promotion rides on that presentation, or the person leaving this time is your best friend and no one else could do her justice, you might start to reconsider that stark 'no'.

Whatever the occasion – even if it's just having the courage to speak up in a meeting at work – the ability to speak clearly and confidently is a great skill to have.

And it is a skill you can learn. All you need are a few tricks of the trade and time to practise. Oh, and this book, of course.

In fact, I'm going to give you one of those tricks of the trade right now, before you've even got to the first chapter:

One of the first things journalists are taught is that every story must cover:

- Who?
- What?
- Why?
- When?
- Where?
- How?

The rule applies equally well to public speaking. We shall be covering these points in detail, but if you remember nothing else, remember to answer all these questions before giving any speech. The rest of the book will show you exactly how they apply.

The Web Tip icon alerts you to where relevant website addresses appear in the text. If you are browsing through the book or specifically looking for website information, these icons will take you straight there.

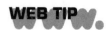

The book is extensively cross referenced and seeing this icon in the margin will help you to find other information within the book relating to the section you are currently reading.

>> p33
How do I end?

To emphasise a good point, this symbol will appear alongside tips for things you should always remember to do.

To highlight a bad point, this symbol will appear alongside things you should always avoid doing.

Throughout the book, true stories have been used to illustrate the points being made in the main text. These are highlighted by the Real Life icon.

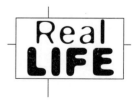

The Jargonbuster margin note is there to highlight and help explain any buzz words or phrases which may crop up.

JARGONBUSTER!
URL (Universal
Resource Locator) is a
web address.

1

THE BASICS

✳ WHY AM I GIVING THIS SPEECH?

✳ WHO AM I TALKING TO?

✳ ALWAYS BE RELEVANT

✳ WHAT AM I TRYING TO ACHIEVE?

A speech is like an iceberg. The part below the surface that no one sees, the preparation of the speech, is 90 per cent of it – but the audience only sees the 10 per cent that is the presentation.

Having been asked to make the speech, you'll be gagging to get on with writing it and won't want to waste any time. STOP! If you've bought this book, you must be willing to do some preparation before committing your eminent wisdom to paper. And this chapter is the most important in the whole book.

Hold your horses until you've really thought through your answers to the next three questions – the holy trinity of public speaking.

WHY AM I GIVING THIS SPEECH?

No one asks you to speak in public without having a good reason. It might be because you're an expert in your field. It might be because you have experienced something that you can convey to an audience. It might be because you're part of a campaign or charitable organisation. Or it might be because the person asking you *thinks* you are one of the above.

The very first thing you need to do is to stop and think about why you've been asked. If you can't answer that question, you may not be the right person to talk and you should bail out right now, before you waste any more time.

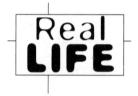

I was once asked to give a presentation about the importance of PR to independent production companies. I was asked because I was then head of PR for a large production group. I didn't research my audience well enough and when I arrived, I discovered they were all tiny companies – one-man bands – and there was no way they could afford an in-house PR. The fault was partly that of the organisers – but I should have done the research. I had to rejig my presentation quickly so that I could say something that would be relevant to the audience.

WHO AM I TALKING TO?

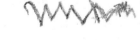

Even if you *are* the right person, talking about the right subject, there is still one potential stumbling block. Are you talking to the right people?

Actually, stop there and rewind. What we should be asking is whether you're pitching the speech at the right level for the audience you've got. If not, it's not the wrong audience, it's the wrong speech. In other words, it's your fault.

The most finely crafted speech, delivered in the clearest style, with the wittiest gags and the most stylish visual backup, will be as dull as ditchwater if you've pitched it wrongly.

TIP

Before you go any further, ask yourself: Why have I been asked to speak? Has whoever asked me explained the speech's purpose?

CHECKLIST OF QUESTIONS

Make sure you know the answers to all the following questions:

Do I know who will be in the audience?
  If not, who can I ask? ❏

How much does the audience know about the subject? ❏

Are they volunteering/paying to listen to me –
  or are they being forced to attend? ❏

How many people will there be? ❏

Will they want facts and statistics or a general message? ❏

What preconceptions might they have about the topic? ❏

Will there be a wide age range? ❏

Will there be a wide range of experience/status? ❏

What will they want to do with the information? ❏

Are they used to listening to verbal presentations? ❏

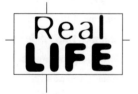

A young advertising executive was asked to talk about effective communication. The event was a trade conference and delegates ranged hugely in age and status. The executive based his entire presentation on children's television of the 1970s. The programmes and advertisements had communicated so effectively with him that they had always stayed with him. Delegates of the same age were amused and gripped by his speech. The older delegates had some idea what he was talking about, although they were usually at work when these programmes were shown. The younger delegates had no idea what he was going on about. They didn't identify with him, they were bored and they got nothing out of the session. He was probably not the right person to speak about effective communication!

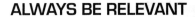

ALWAYS BE RELEVANT

If you were asked to talk to schoolchildren about road safety, you would probably keep the information to the bare essentials. You might take them into the playground and demonstrate how to cross the road or how to use a pelican crossing.

A talk to their parents about the same issue would be much more hard hitting. The audience would probably stay indoors, sitting down, and you might discuss specific accident blackspots in the area, while debating what improvements could be made.

Get these round the wrong way and the children would be bored and frightened, while the adults would feel silly and patronised.

A talk to local policemen, again about road safety, would be different altogether. You would probably be even more specific, more hard hitting and you would use more statistics and examples. You would also need to tell the policemen how to educate the children and parents of the area.

Coincidentally, the policemen may also be parents but, in this context, they are expecting a professional and businesslike approach.

Find out what the audience expects of you – always tailor your speech to the right context and never patronise your audience!

DO AN INTERNET SEARCH TOO. Most larger companies now have their own websites, including recent press releases, financial information, etc. By reading this, you'll be able to find out their current priorities.

If you don't know their web address (otherwise known as a URL), try guessing! It's not as daft as it might sound. Try typing www.[nameofcompany].co.uk or www.[nameofcompany].com.

For example, if you wanted to find out about Tesco, you would type **'www.tesco.com'**. And you would be right! If that doesn't work, try to track it down through one of the search engines, such as **www.google.com** or **www.yahoo.co.uk** (see chapter 2 for more on using the internet for research).

URL (Universal Resource Locator) is a web address. Usually looks like this: www.nameofcompany.co.uk or www.nameofcompany.com.

http:// You sometimes see these symbols at the beginning of a web

TIP
If you're speaking to the employees of a company, phone in advance and ask the human resources department for more information.

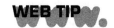

>> p. 16
Flesh it out with research

JARGONBUSTER!
http:// These symbols simply tell the computer that the address is for a web page.

TIP
Most browsers don't actually need you to type http:// at the beginning of the web address – they will add it automatically. But it won't hurt if you do type it. It's often included to help readers recognise it as a web address, especially if the address doesn't include the letters www.

address. They simply tell the computer that the address is for a web page. The letters 'http' actually stand for Hypertext Transfer Protocol, which is the method the internet uses to send web pages.

www.bazza.com This bit is the address itself – the name of the computer that holds the web server that hosts the site.

/sj/humour If you see forward slashes and other words after the main site address, they are simply directing you to the actual pages you want to see. They are usually a good thing because they save you having to find your way around a site that may be unfamiliar.

htm Some web addresses end with the letters 'htm' or 'html'. This stands for Hypertext Markup Language and is the code in which web pages are written. If the web address doesn't end like this, the computer will usually use a default document.

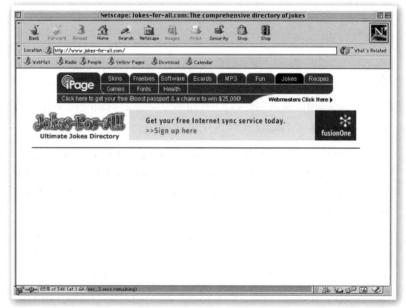

ILLUSTRATION 1   Screen grab of search page of jokesforall.com

WHAT AM I TRYING TO ACHIEVE?

You know why they've asked you and you know who you're talking to. Now we can really get to work. I'll be referring to this section right through this book, so you might as well concentrate while you're here.

What do you want to achieve from this speech? To help you answer, let's break it down into two elements:

1. What's my Objective?

2. What do I want the End Result to be?

At first, these might seem to be the same, but let's have a closer look:

OBJECTIVES
There are several possible objectives for a speech, but they usually fall into one of the following:

● to inform

● to prompt an action

● to provoke emotion

● to entertain

● to promote discussion

If you are asked to speak at a wedding, you will be expected to entertain. You will be speaking to friends and family, to whom you would normally speak informally, even though a wedding is a fairly formal occasion.

If you are so incensed about road safety in your area that you decide to set up an action group, you will need to inspire other parents to join you. Your presentation to them must make them share your anger and prompt them to do something about it.

A presentation to your board of directors about sales figures for the last quarter will mainly need to inform. The information itself should be enough. Forget jokes and emotional declarations.

But if those sales figures were poor, you'll have to inspire the sales team, when you get back to the office. You might need to scold or cajole the team – probably a bit of both. This will be much more informal and personal and with much more emotion.

END RESULTS

Once you've worked out your Objective, you can get more detailed and personal, and work out what your End Result should be.

CHECKLIST

It's easy to get carried away dreaming about what you want your End Result to be. Ask yourself, is my End Result. . .

Definable? ❏

Reasonable? ❏

Possible? ❏

Imagine you've delivered your speech. Everything's gone really well and members of the opposite sex are falling at your feet with admiration for your immense speaking talents. What should happen next? (Apart from picking out the cutest of your new fans and taking them for a drink, I mean.)

Do you want the audience to do something? What? Do you want them to apply their new-found knowledge? How? Your Objective might be a bit airy-fairy, but your End Result should get down to specifics.

If you have the End Result clear in your mind, you will be more likely to achieve it.

Objective: To inspire fellow parents to join me in a fight for road safety improvements in the village.

End Result: The parents will sign my petition and write to the council. They will be inspired enough to come to another meeting next week.

If I had simply worked out my Objective, I'd have some idea where I was going. But I'd have no way of knowing exactly how to pitch it, nor could I measure how successful the speech was because I hadn't worked out the End Result.

Have another look at the End Result for the road safety campaign. You'll see that it was all three things required of any End Result. It was:

Definable = I can look at the petition and see how many people have signed. And how many turn up next time.

Reasonable = I'm not asking for the moon on a stick. People are busy and I can't expect everyone to devote hours and hours to this. But they can sign a petition, write a letter and turn up next week.

Possible = It's important to note that my End Result wasn't to improve road safety. That's because it's simply not possible for this meeting to achieve that. Only the council can authorise the money and the work.

TIP

Write down your Objective and End Result on a piece of paper. Stick it up somewhere obvious while you're writing your presentation.

SUMMARY

You should now have answered the questions we set at the beginning of the chapter. Let's recap:

Why have I been asked to speak?

Think about the person who asked you – are you clear about their agenda?

Who am I talking to?

Think about who is in the audience and how you can find out more about them, including their needs, expertise and expectations.

What do I want to achieve?

Set your Objective and your End Result. These will be the solid foundations on which you build your presentation.

2

PLANNING AND

STRUCTURE

✳ MAKE YOURSELF A MIND MAP

✳ TURN IT INTO A ROUTE MAP

✳ FLESH IT OUT WITH RESEARCH

You're already on your way. You've established your Objective and worked out from that what you want your End Result to be. You know your audience and what they expect from you.

But even setting your Objective probably got you thinking about dozens and dozens of associated subheadings and topics. You know they're not all relevant to this audience – they might be too far reaching – and they're not all relevant to your End Result. But how on earth do you decide what to include and what to leave out?

There will probably be a million thoughts milling around in your head. First of all, don't panic. All you have to do is think through your presentation in a logical manner and there are a number of ways to help you do this.

Planning is the key to constructing a good speech.

MAKE YOURSELF A MIND MAP

In order to know where we're travelling, we all need a map. And as you're taking the audience on a journey through your topic, they, and you, need exactly that.

There are three main steps to drawing up your map, and you can run through these either by yourself or in a brainstorming session.

There are several ways of drawing up your plan, but my favourite is to create a Mind Map.

If your subject is new to you, or requires a lot of thought, you might want to kick the creation of your Mind Map off with a brainstorming session. Some of the brainstorms I've been to were both fascinating and intellectually stimulating. Others were less of a brain*storm* and more a brain *damp breeze*. There's a trick to them.

1 Only invite a maximum of eight people, unless they know each other very well (large groups can intimidate people and kill creativity).

2 Invite people who know the topic well and some who don't know it at all (they'll bring no baggage and preconceived ideas with them).

3 Provide water, tea, coffee, wine, beer, nibbles – anything that will make people more comfortable.

4 Run through the reason for calling the brainstorm.

5 Appoint a manager to channel suggestions and make sure everyone gets a say.

6 Appoint a writer to scribble down suggestions on a whiteboard, flip chart or Post-it notes, which are then stuck to a wall. You choose what method.

7 Open the floodgates.

8 Don't stop until you've exhausted all possibilities. Only when you've got a long list should you start to decide on which ideas are the best.

Brainstorms are supposed to be free-for-alls, but it might help to apply a few simple rules.

TIP

When you're working out the structure of your talk, take the Objective, End Result and audience as your compass and you won't steer far off course.

TIP

Listen to all the ideas at a brainstorming session but make sure someone is in charge to keep the meeting on course.

- Business or social hierarchy is left at the door. Everyone is equal.

- No one can rubbish anyone else's ideas.

- All ideas must be shared, even if they seem stupid.

- All ideas must be written down.

- Managers can't try to influence anyone's thinking.

Whether you decide to make your Mind Map yourself, or you want to enlist other people to help you, there are just three simple stages. Using a piece of paper, a flip chart, a whiteboard or Post-it notes, as suggested above:

IDENTIFY YOUR CENTRAL MESSAGE This will normally be your Objective, or a word or phrase closely associated with it. Write it in the middle of the page.

IDENTIFY SECONDARY POINTS These are the subheadings, which in turn suggest their own subheadings.

ALL AROUND THE CENTRAL MESSAGE, draw arrows to your secondary points. Where the secondary points suggest further points, continue the arrows out like a ladder. When you've exhausted the possibilities,

LEAVE THINGS OUT These are the bits you dream up as secondary points and then decide to cross out. Return to your Objective, End Result and audience profile and consider which of your points are vital and which beyond the scope of your speech. Cross out anything that doesn't fit in. Be ruthless!

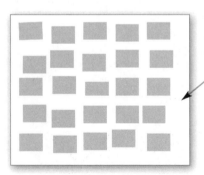

First board

Sticky notes with brainstormed ideas listed at random.

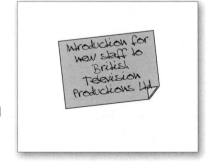

Second board

Central message.

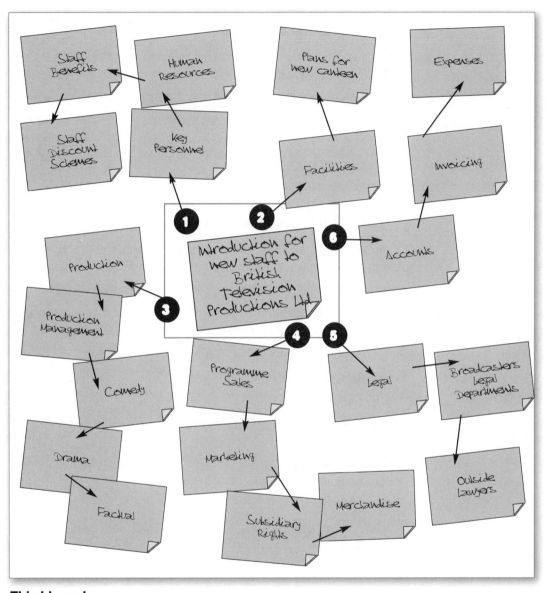

Third board

Secondary ideas sorted into a Mind Map around the central message.

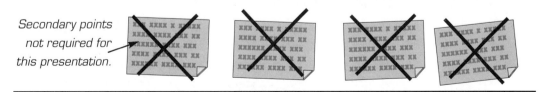

Secondary points not required for this presentation.

ILLUSTRATION 2:   Stages in planning a Mind Map

CHECKLIST

When deciding what to include, ask yourself the following questions:

What will they expect me to cover first? ❑

Which points will best pave the way
    to explain my later points? ❑

TURN IT INTO A ROUTE MAP

You've done your Mind Map, so you know which points are in and which are out. But at the moment, the bones of your speech skeleton are scattered all over the page.

It's all down there, but now you've got to meld those scattered bones into a sensible structure. How?

As you think these through, it will probably become obvious that some points need to come before others.

If your Route Map isn't obvious, try jotting down each point onto a separate card and shuffling them about until you get the right structure.

When you have found the most logical route through your topic, identify the key Stepping Stones (probably the secondary points you established above).

It might help to think of this stage like a book, with your Objective, or central message, as the title of the book and your key points, or Stepping Stones, as the chapter headings.

FLESH IT OUT WITH RESEARCH

Now you have the skeleton of your speech, you need to put some flesh on those bones and fill in what you're going to say about each Stepping Stone. The first thing to do is to tackle any necessary research. The internet has revolutionised research: almost everything you need to know about anything is out there on the World Wide Web.

We touched on this subject in chapter 1 when we discussed researching the audience, but let's take a more detailed look at the vast resource that is the World Wide Web.

>> p. 13
**What am I trying
to achieve?**

SEARCH ENGINES

Unless you know exactly what you're looking for and you know the URL of the site, start with one of the search engines or directories (see below).

There are dozens of major search sites. They create their own indexes which are constantly updated by special programs called spiders. A search engine will ask you for a key word to search. When you've typed it in, a kind of electronic gopher rushes out and scours the Web for that word. It will display a list of sites containing the word or words you were asking for.

JARGONBUSTER!

**A search engine is a
huge index of websites.**

Different sites have programmed their gophers in different ways, so it's worth trying the same word in a few search engines – you'll probably get different results.

DIRECTORIES

As an alternative to the search engines, you might want to use a directory, such as Yahoo! These are lists of web pages, sorted into categories. You *can* search most directory sites using a key word, but the best way is to use the category links. Scroll down the page a bit until you can see them all. Then click through sub-categories until you find what you want.

SOME OF THE BEST SEARCH ENGINES

Yahoo! UK and Ireland	www.yahoo.co.uk
Excite	www.excite.com
Lycos UK	www.lycos.co.uk
UK Plus	www.ukplus.co.uk
AltaVista	www.altavista.digital.com
Infoseek	www.infoseek.co.uk
Ask	www.ask.co.uk

(this one works slightly differently: you key in a question, such as 'Where can I find out about labradors on the Web?')

SEARCH TIPS

The simplest way of searching is to click the cursor into the textbox, type in a single word and then click on the 'search' button. You will then be presented with a list of sites that match your keyword.

DO use capital letters if you want to find capital letters. So if you want to find out about London, type 'London', not 'LONDON' or 'london'. For ordinary words, such as 'poetry', simply use lower case.

DO put quote marks around the word to find a phrase. So 'love poems' will search for love poems and not just 'love' or 'poems'.

DO use + and – (a hyphen will do). If you are looking for, say, hotels in Chicago, try typing: 'hotels + Chicago'. But if you're trying to find out other things about Chicago and don't want to know about hotels, try typing: 'Chicago – hotels'.

JARGONBUSTER!
Favourites/bookmarks:
most web browsers
allow you to save
website addresses to a
special file.

Given the vast amount of information on the Web, refining your search makes sense in order to avoid ploughing through thousands of sites.

FAVOURITES OR BOOKMARKS

If a site looks interesting, add it to the Favourites or Bookmarks section of your web browser. That way you'll be able to find it again easily. If you're using Internet Explorer this facility is called 'Favourites'. Netscape, another popular browser, calls it 'Bookmarks'.

When you've done a search, you can also add the results page to your Favourites list and come back to it in the future.

When you've found a site you think you might want to come back to, go to the menu bar at the top of the screen, click on 'Favourites' or 'Bookmarks' and follow the straightforward steps.

Then, when you want to retrieve the site, go back in and click on the address. It'll whizz you straight to your chosen site.

When the search engine gives you a list of results, click on a title to go through to the site it has suggested. Don't worry, you won't get lost – you can always click 'Back' in the top left of your computer screen.

BUSINESS SEARCHES

If you're looking for a particular business or service, try the online versions of *Scoot* or *Yellow Pages* (Yell).

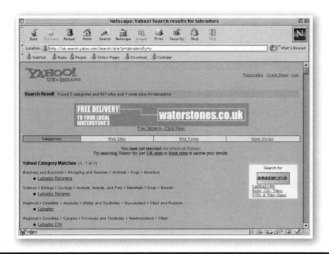

IllUSTRATION 3:   A typical search engine results page will look like this

Yell can be found at **www.yell.co.uk**

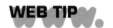

Scoot is at **www.scoot.co.uk**

Both sites allow you to search by business name or type and by location. They will present you with a list of company names, addresses and telephone numbers. If the company has a website or email address, the site will usually include a link to these as well.

OTHER USEFUL SOURCES ON THE INTERNET
The trick to getting the most out of the internet is to think laterally.

If there is a trade body, charity or society associated with your subject, take a look at their website. Most carry useful background information about their subject, either under obvious category headings or under the heading FAQ.

The Government has pledged to get as many services online as it can, as quickly as it can. Government departments already have their own sites. While they're almost universally ugly and utilitarian, they contain useful statistics, press releases and reports.

Local councils also have websites, which can be useful for local information.

Most of these sites have URLs ending in the suffix '.gov.uk', for example, the website of the Ministry of Agriculture, Fisheries and Food is **www.maff.gov.uk**.

JARGONBUSTER!
FAQ (Frequently Asked Questions): a document containing some of the most commonly asked questions, plus answers. A useful resource if you're new to a topic.

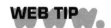

You can get the URLs for all government departments and local councils at www.open.gov.uk – a really useful directory which covers all government bodies, including organisations such as the Association of Police Authorities and ACAS (the Advisory, Conciliation and Arbitration Service).

The national newspapers have been mystifyingly slow to catch on to the potential of the internet. However, most of them now have sites up and running, with useful archive sections, containing old news reports and features. By far the best is the one for the *Guardian* – **www.guardianunlimited.co.uk**. The *Financial Times* website, **www.ft.com**, is also an impressive resource.

BBC Online is also a brilliant resource. The news service is pretty good and the site has lots of other sections, covering subjects such as food, gardening, health etc. Find it at **www.bbc.co.uk**.

The trade paper for your subject might also have a site, e.g. **www.businessweek.com**; **www.produxion.com** (TV/radio trade site).

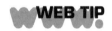

For an absolutely mind-bogglingly vast directory of website addresses for newspapers around the world, visit the Internet Public Library at www.ipl.org. The UK section includes links to around a hundred national and local newspapers.

Other sites you might find useful include:

- Dow Jones: **www.dowjones.com**
- Teletext: **www.teletext.co.uk**
- The History Channel.com: **www.historychannel.com**
- The World Wide Web Virtual Library: **www.vlib.org**
- Librarians' Index to the internet: **www.lii.org**
- Free internet Encyclopedia: **www.clever.net/cam/encyclopedia**
- The Living Encyberpedia: **www.encyberpedia.com**
- Ref Desk: **www.refdesk.com**

For more advice on research, together with links to dozens of features on the subject, try the US site **www.cs.cmu.edu/afs/cs.cmu.edu/mleone/web/how-to**.

OTHER RESEARCH TOOLS

LIBRARIES. Books are valuable research tools but libraries nowadays also have video or audio tapes and CD-ROMs.

NEWSPAPERS AND MAGAZINES. Apart from the resources held on the internet, there are other ways of looking into the archives of a publication. Many produce their own CD-ROMs, such as the *Daily Mail*'s excellent one. Some trade papers maintain their own archive, while others will be held by associated trade bodies. Some publications even issue annual indexes, which help you find your way round the year's issues. Call the publisher's office for information. The British Library Newspaper Division at Colindale in London holds copies of all main magazines and newspapers. These can be ordered ahead and may be viewable either in their original printed form, or, more likely, on microfiche or similar.

TRADE BODIES, CHARITIES AND COMMERCIAL ORGANISATIONS. Most of these now have their own websites, crammed with useful information. However, if you don't have internet access or your relevant organisation still lives in the Dark Ages, you may be able to access their information in other ways. Some may operate a library, or produce special publications, mailed to members or other interested parties.

SUMMARY

You have developed your thoughts and gathered them up into a coherent structure. Let's recap:

Your Mind Map ...

Help yourself to identify what should be included
– and what you should leave out!

Your Route Map

Take the bones of your ideas and build them into a solid skeleton for your presentation.

Your research

Get to grips with research, including the internet – the library that comes direct to your desktop.

3

DECIDING ON
THE WORDS

* SCRIPTS VERSUS CUE CARDS

* HOW TO START

* HOW TO CARRY ON

* HOW TO FINISH BIG

* POLISHING THE SPEECH

Hooray! I'm delighted to tell you that, believe it or not, you've now done most of the hard work. Preparing a speech or presentation is a bit like decorating a room. The bit that you're itching to get to is choosing colours, slapping paint over the walls and putting all your belongings and new toys back into the room. But if you jump to that stage without first removing the old wallpaper, washing the walls and sanding down, the finish will be shoddy and the cracks will soon show. As it is in DIY, so it is in public speaking.

But you've now done all that boring preparation and you've got to the colour-chart stage – the stage where you pull the whole thing together and start writing your speech.

SCRIPTS VERSUS CUE CARDS

If you're not used to speaking in public, there's a huge temptation to write the whole speech out in full and simply read it out from your prepared script.

On the plus side, you'll never be stuck for a word, you'll never have to improvise and you'll know exactly where you are at any one time.

You could do it this way – many people do. But I would suggest that reading from a script is like riding your bike with stabilisers. You'll still move forward and you will, indeed, be safe from falling down, but you'll be restricted in what you can do. Remember the day you took the stabilisers off your bike? It was exhilarating, wasn't it? Suddenly you could whizz round corners and weave in and out of obstacles. You were free!

So I would urge you to remove the stabilisers of the script and move on to the freewheeling excitement (OK, maybe that's stretching the metaphor a touch too far!) of cue cards. Let's run through this approach and then you can make your choice.

Cue cards are

- ● easier to handle

- ● less likely to get damaged

- ● smaller and thicker – so it's less noticeable if you're shaking

You *can* jump straight from your Route Map to your cue cards. To create your Route Map, you identified your key points, the main stepping stones of your speech. These should now form the basis for your cue cards.

But if you're not a frequent speaker, I would suggest that instead of jumping from Route Map to cue card, you're probably better off getting there in three easy steps.

STEP 1: CREATE YOUR TEXT

Taking your Route Map and a clean pad of paper or new computer wordprocessing document, note down your Stepping Stones, or key points, one on each page. Under each key point, list the subsidiary points that you identified when you made your Mind Map.

Keep filling in, using your expertise and the research you've done, until you've roughed out the whole speech. Throughout this process, keep looking at the Objective and End Result that you wrote out and pinned up nearby.

STEP 2: TURN YOUR TEXT INTO A SCRIPT

In step 1, you pulled together all the information into a coherent whole. But you haven't yet got a speech.

There is a big difference between the written word and the spoken word. (Unless you're *Trainspotting* author Irvine Welsh, in which case there's no difference at all.) But generally, if you read out a passage directly from a book, exactly as it's written, you will find it sounds stilted and odd.

>> p. 38

Polishing your speech **Read the tips in 'Polishing your speech', for more about the differences between written and spoken English.**

At this stage, you should also start thinking about the visual aids you might want to use to support your presentation – you might note these cues in your script. (See opposite for the difference between a text page and a script.)

STEP 3: TURN YOUR SCRIPT INTO CUE CARDS

Using your main points as your framework, this is where you will distil your script down into key words or phrases.

If your speech is quite simple and short, you should be able to put one of your Stepping Stones, or key points, on each cue card. Write this in big letters and then add your key words and phrases.

But don't cram things onto the cards! If you've got a lot to say and only a few Stepping Stones, break things down a little further and devote a new card to each of your subheadings. The trick is to keep the information on each card to a minimum.

Number your cards, just in case you drop them on the floor! And move your thumb down the card as you move through the points. Then, when you look up to speak, you won't have lost your place.

TEXT PAGE

I would like to take this opportunity to welcome you all as new members of staff at British Television Productions Limited. For those of you who do not know me, my name is Joan Brown and I am the director of human resources.

The purpose of this meeting is to give you all a quick rundown of the different departments in the company and to explain how they relate to each other. You will be able to see how you fit into the bigger picture and, hopefully, it will help you to understand who your colleagues are and what their role entails. I am going to ask you to look at some slides, including photographs of the most senior staff. As you can see, BTP is run by an executive committee of eight people. This is the chief executive, Peter Hammond . . .

SCRIPT PAGE

(WELCOME)

For those of you who don't know me, I'm Joan Brown and I'm the director of human resources.

The purpose of this meeting is to give you a quick rundown of the different departments in the company and to explain how they relate to each other.

(DISTRIBUTE LEAFLETS SHOWING COMPANY STRUCTURE)

As you can see from the chart, BTP is run by an executive committee of eight people . . .

(TRIGGER FIRST SLIDE)

ILLUSTRATION 4: Sample text page compared to sample script page

CUE CARD 1

(Welcome)

Introduce self

Purpose: rundown of different departments

Explain slides

CUE CARD 2

(Distribute handouts showing company structure)

Explain executive committee

(Trigger first slide)

CUE CARD 3

Peter Hammond profile

(Trigger second slide)

Identify executive committee members

CUE CARD 4

(Trigger third slide)

Identify the human resources team

Move on to staff benefits

CUE CARD 5

(Trigger fourth slide)

Talk about new sports club

Explain staff discount schemes

CUE CARD 6

Explain facilities available to staff

(Trigger fifth slide)

Relate plans for new canteen

ILLUSTRATION 5:   Part of your speech as it might appear on cue cards

You really should trust your memory – you will remember much more than you think.

If you're still not sure you can trust your memory, do two sets of key words – a minimum version and a more thorough one. Then you can practise with each. If you feel a bit nervous, use the more thorough version, but you may well find that you remember perfectly and that you speak more naturally with the minimum version.

The reason I recommend the cue card approach is because I believe it gives *just enough* freedom. It frees you from the constraints of a written script, making your words sound fresher, more genuine and more conversational. But, unlike learning a speech by heart, it gives you a little support and, if you're getting off the point, it will take you straight back to your Objective.

TIP

Note the points at which you want to introduce any props or visual aids, but do this in a different colour. You'll be able to see it coming and this will prevent you from saying 'start slide show' out loud, by mistake!

HOW TO START

You've already decided on what your first point should be, and where you're going from there. Now you need to decide how to start saying it!

Beginnings are hugely important. This is the point at which you set the scene for the whole of the presentation. The audience will be at their most receptive and full of curiosity. It's at this point that they're going to decide whether they like you; whether you're going to be interesting; and whether they made the right decision in coming along at all.

Grab their attention now and they're more likely to stay with you throughout the speech. Lose them at the beginning and you'll never get them back.

BEGINNINGS SHOULD:
- have impact
- have authority: show the audience you know your subject
- show awareness of the audience's needs, expectations and interests
- be appropriate: don't tell a dodgy joke to an audience of professionals expecting a political speech, and don't let it jar with the rest of the speech

DON'T stare at an empty page, agonising about how to start. Write the main body of the speech first. So feel free to skip the beginning and come back to it later. You'll probably then find the beginning writes itself.

The key to a good intro is simply this: **give the audience a reason to listen.** There are several ways of doing this. Here are some examples:

1 Promise them something they want

I'm going to tell you about a product that will save you time and money AND improve your love life.

2 Tell them it's going to be short and simple

I know you've given up your free evening to be here tonight, so I'm only going to make three short points.

3 Tell them a story

We stand on a lonely, windswept point on the northern shore of France. The air is soft, but forty years ago at this moment, the air was filled with the crack of rifle fire and the roar of cannon. At dawn, on the morning of the 6th of June 1944, 225 Rangers jumped off the British landing-craft and ran to the bottom of these cliffs.

Ronald Reagan, 6 June 1984, taken from *The Penguin Book of Twentieth-Century Speeches.*

4 Create an image

Before I came here tonight, I went to visit little Johnny Smith in hospital. Johnny – a boy we've often seen trotting off to school – was lying in a hospital bed, fighting for his life, hooked up to all kinds of monitors and machines.

5 Shock them

I speak to you as a man who fifty years and nine days ago had no name, no hope, no future and was known only by his number, A, 70713.

Auschwitz survivor Elie Wiesel, 27 January 1995, taken from *The Penguin Book of Twentieth-Century Speeches.*

6 Make 'em laugh

The first time I took Tracey out on a date, I went to her house to pick her up. Her dad said she was just putting the finishing touches to her makeup. And then he said: 'Fancy a game of chess?'

7 Ask them questions

Do you find yourself constantly struggling because you haven't got enough time or money? Do you want to make your life easier?

All the above examples give the audience a reason for listening. You have made the speech directly relevant to them and so they want to know more.

HOW TO CARRY ON

You have your Route Map, so let the audience in on the secret; tell them where they're going. This isn't a magical mystery tour – the less the audience knows, the more time they're going to spend wondering, just when you want their attention.

Think about the times you have listened to speeches. If the speaker was boring you were drifting into a daydream, or trying to guess how long they were going to bang on because you were hungry/needed a wee/couldn't wait to get to the bar, etc.

Tell the audience where you are taking them.

So when preparing the speech, make sure you've answered all their possible questions.

And don't forget to present these in a positive light. Make the topic relevant, make yourself attractive to them, and tell them you're not going to speak for long. Today, we're so used to watching 60-second commercials. Airtime sales experts carefully place ads in programmes that the target market will be watching. So the ad is aimed at *you*, it's also visually gorgeous, may contain great music, *and* it gets its message across. Phew! How can you possibly compete?

Well, you *can* compete, because your speech is targeted directly at the dozen or couple of hundred people in the room. You've got something interesting to say and if you put it across properly, they'll listen.

Once you've answered their subconscious questions, move through the presentation by simply linking your different points.

Research has shown that most people have short attention spans. If you're speaking for 40 minutes, they'll start off listening intently and their interest will wane until it reaches its lowest ebb about 30 minutes into the speech. Then they'll sense the end is near and they'll perk up again.

But they'll listen more intently and more consistently to four ten-minute speeches. So why not try to break up your speech into shorter bursts, using visuals, a show of hands or some other stunt? You might even think back to those commercials and give your audience four five-minute breaks instead of one 15-minute break.

See 'Polishing your speech', for more tips on how to retain the audience's attention.

HOW TO FINISH BIG

In many ways, the ending is even more important than the opening. If you start well, keep them listening throughout the presentation and then limp to a sad little halt, that poor ending will undo all the good work you did at the beginning.

The ending is a chance to recap and should be the climax of your speech. When you are ending your speech:

DO pull people together.

>> p38

Polishing your speech

DO reinforce the message.

DO call the audience to action.

There are a number of ways to ensure that your ending will prove a fitting climax. Here are some options:

LEARN IT BY HEART

Your finale should trip off the tongue and sound like you mean it. This is not a time for stumbling over your words. Make sure it's smooth and delivered with confidence.

GIVE ADDED VALUE

Today, we've looked at eight main points – People, Response, Organisation, Growth, Results, Excellence, Service and Sustainability. Put them all together, and we have PROGRESS.

Ending with a punchy and memorable little message should certainly help everyone to remember what it was you were talking about.

ADD DRAMA OR EMOTION

Above all, we give thanks for the life of a woman I am so proud to be able to call my sister: the unique, the complex, the extraordinary and irreplaceable Diana, whose beauty, both internal and external, will never be extinguished from our minds.

Earl Spencer, at the funeral of Diana, Princess of Wales, 6 September 1997, taken from *The Penguin Book of Twentieth-Century Speeches.*

Fortunately, not everyone will have to give such an address, but an emotional or highly dramatic sting in your speech's tail will certainly make it more memorable.

GIVE AN IMPORTANT FACT

As you know, our main competitor has just been taken over. I've found out that the new parent company has one million pounds to invest in researching new markets. If we're to remain market leader, we need to act now.

Something which is of great importance to your audience will have the same effect as a dramatic or emotionally charged ending.

PROVIDE A PAY-OFF YOU SET UP AT THE BEGINNING

So I'd like to say a special thank-you to Tracey for becoming my wife. I think you'll all agree that she makes a beautiful bride – and that she's really achieved something today: all her makeup done to perfection and only 10 minutes late at the church!

A pay-off line provides a neat, well-rounded ending.

CHECKLIST

Have I told the audience

my topic: what I'm talking about?	❏
my reason for speaking?	❏
the limits – what I can and can't tackle in this presentation?	❏
the time allowed for questions at the end	❏

JOHN F KENNEDY'S INAUGURAL ADDRESS, 20 JANUARY 1961

BEGINNING: Welcome … we observe today not a victory of party, but a celebration of freedom symbolising an end, as well as a beginning, signifying renewal, as well as change. For I have sworn before you and Almighty God the same solemn oath our forebears prescribed nearly a century and three quarters ago.

The world is very different now. For man holds in his mortal hands the power to abolish all forms of human poverty and all forms of human life. And yet the same revolutionary beliefs for which our forebears fought are still at issue around the globe, the belief that the rights of man come not from the generosity of the state, but from the hand of God …

ENDING: … And so, my fellow Americans, ask not what your country can do for you; ask what you can do for your country.

My fellow citizens of the world: ask not what America will do for you, but what together we can do for the freedom of man.

Finally, whether you are citizens of America or citizens of the world, ask of us the same high standards of strength and sacrifice which we ask of you. With a good conscience our only sure reward, with history the final judge of our deeds, let us go forth to lead the land we love, asking His blessing and His help, but knowing that here on earth God's work must truly be our own.

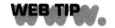 **For John F Kennedy's complete speech, visit** www.bartleby.com

ILLUSTRATION 6:   Beginnings and endings of two famous speeches

MARTIN LUTHER KING'S 'I HAVE A DREAM' SPEECH, 28 AUGUST 1963

BEGINNING: I am happy to join with you today in what will go down in history as the greatest demonstration for freedom in the history of our nation.

Fivescore years ago, a great American, in whose symbolic shadow we stand today, signed the Emancipation Proclamation. This momentous decree came as a great beacon light of hope to millions of Negro slaves who had been seared in the flames of withering injustice. It came as a joyous daybreak to end the long night of their captivity.

But one hundred years later, the Negro still is not free. One hundred years later, the life of the Negro is still sadly cripped by the manacles of segregation and the chains of discrimination. One hundred years later, the Negro lives on a lonely island of poverty in the midst of a vast ocean of material prosperity. One hundred years later, the Negro is still languished in the corners of American society and finds himself an exile in his own land. And so we've come here today to dramatise a shameful condition …

ENDING: This is our hope. This is the faith that I go back to the South with. With this faith we will be able to hew out of the mountain of despair a stone of hope. With this faith we will be able to transform the jangling discords of our nation into a beautiful symphony of brotherhood. With this faith, we will be able to work together, to pray together, to struggle together, to go to jail together, to stand up for freedom together, knowing that we will be free one day. This will be the day, this will be the day when all of God's children will be able to sing with new meaning

'My country, tis of thee, sweet land of liberty, of thee I sing'

… And when this happens, when we allow freedom to ring, when we let it ring from every village and every hamlet, from every state and every city, we will be able to speed up that day when all of God's children, black men and white men, Jews and Gentiles, Protestants and Catholics, will be able to join hands and sing in the words of the old Negro spiritual: 'Free at last! Free at last! Thank God Almighty, we are free at last.'

For the full text of Martin Luther King's speech, visit www.stanford.edu/group/King/

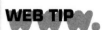
WEB TIP

POLISHING YOUR SPEECH

Right, you've got the words down on paper and in your mind – and in the right order too! But don't rush off to deliver the presentation just yet. To make the difference between a good enough speech and a really good speech, you need to get out the literary Mr Sheen and polish up your English.

Here are a few suggestions that might help.

GET CHATTY

As we discussed above, spoken English is very different from written English. Listen to real conversations (a great excuse for nosy Parkers). Next time you're on the bus or waiting in a queue, listen to the words and sentence structure people use.

You will find that their speech patterns are full of abbreviations, such as 'you'll', 'didn't', 'wouldn't', etc., and they break off in the middle of sentences and use 'incorrect' grammar.

In your speech, you need to find a healthy balance between the boring correctness of written English and the muddled informality of having a chat.

 DO read your draft speech out loud enough times to get comfortable with it. If you're using cue cards, this should be easy. If you've decided to ignore my good advice and read from a script, then you'll find it harder. Don't stick too closely to the written word – let your natural speech patterns come out. It will be much more interesting for your audience.

If you rush the audience, or blind them with long words, they'll be too busy worrying about the bits they missed to concentrate on the later pearls of wisdom.

Think about the three key differences between written and spoken words:

WRITTEN	SPOKEN
at reader's own pace	at speaker's pace
can be re-read	heard only once
can be read in any order	only heard in the order it's presented

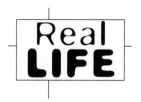

Although he's hardly read these days, W W Jacobs is one of my family's favourite authors. His comic short stories were hugely popular at the beginning of the 20th century and he was admired by many better-known writers, including P G Wodehouse.

One of Jacobs's charms lies in his ability to convey normal speech patterns and dialect on the written page.

Take this extract from the opening chapter of his book Deep Waters*:*

'A sailorman – said the night-watchman musingly – a sailorman is like a fish, he is safest when 'e is at sea. When a fish comes ashore it is in for trouble, and so is a sailorman. One poor chap I knew 'ardly ever came ashore without getting married; and when he was found out there was no less than six wimmen in the court all taking away 'is character at once.'

Jacobs's writing was unusual for its time – he was a middle-class man himself, but a shrewd observer of the speech and language of all kinds of people. This 'chatty' style is easy to read and, in the above extract, we learn more about the night-watchman than could be conveyed in pages and pages of description.

DO avoid boring, passive words and phrases and go for exciting, active, thrilling language.

DO say, 'Our approach gets results fast! We could boost your productivity by a third in just six months.'

DON'T say, 'It has been found that our training course can improve productivity by an average of 33 per cent within six months.'

The same goes for phrases – make sure you keep them dynamic!

When you are thinking about your style, try reading the tabloid newspapers. If you're a snob about newspapers, you're in for a shock. It's the tabloids that are the true masters at conveying complicated stories in the simplest, most dynamic language. Sometimes they use terrible 'journalese', but ignore this and try to break down how they've put the story across. You might want to compare the same story in different types of newspapers.

DON'T SAY	DO SAY
you might want to	you should
I think you should	you should
can we think about	let's think about
shouldn't we try to	we must
may	can
could	can
might	will

USE THE RIGHT WORDS

Remember that words convey different emotions. Think about what buttons you want to press for your audience and use words that feel appropriate.

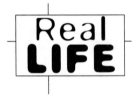

As I wrote those words, I was casting around for a good example to illustrate what I meant. My partner works for one of the big food chains, so a copy of The Grocer *magazine happened to be lying on the coffee table. I just opened it at a random page and found an ad for the launch of a new range of chicken ready-meals.*

The ad said in big letters: 'Quality chicken. Altogether more tempting.'

It went on: 'With more thought for food, Birds Eye have once again made chicken altogether more tempting with the launch of two delicious and original dishes – Thai Chicken and Honey and Mustard Chicken.'

The copywriters and product developers have really thought about what the average household is looking for and they've pulled out all the right words to get that message across.

Health scares have rocked our confidence in the safety of meat, so 'quality' is there to reassure. But it's food, so it must be 'tempting' – a ready-meal is a bit of a treat, not something most families have every day. And so it goes on – the food is 'delicious' and 'original' – it's got to taste good, and how many home cooks are bored with preparing the same food, week in, week out?

Another example:

My newspaper property section carries an ad today that warns:

'Prepare to be converted. Nightingale Court features a range of large, elegant apartments of unreserved luxury set in two landmark Victorian listed buildings in extensively landscaped mature grounds. These magnificent apartments combine traditional Victorian architecture with modern design and materials, blending the very best of old and new.'

Talk about pushing the right buttons! The developers know their customer – probably a well-off but busy commuter. He likes the character of older properties but hasn't the time or skills to do up an old wreck. He wants the best home, for the minimum fuss. He wants to put his deckchair outside on occasion, but he doesn't want to do the gardening. A different kind of buyer might be looking for a cosy family home – not our man! He wants to impress guests, so his home needs to be 'magnificent'.

Without realising he's being manipulated, our buyer will be very interested in this particular property.

Keep your Objective in mind all the time.

You can make your speech even more relevant to your audience by choosing the right words. Go back to your Objective. Is your speech about selling a product that can save the audience time? Use snappy words; appeal to their busy, stressed lives. Is it about asking them to join a campaign? Appeal to their emotions with warm, powerful words.

DO jot down what you want to say and then use a thesaurus to find a more exciting way of saying it. For example, if you jotted down 'Your profits will increase', the thesaurus offers you all kinds of interesting alternatives for 'increase': amplify, heighten, inflate, snowball, magnify, boost, multiply, escalate, enlarge, proliferate … there is plenty of choice.

THINK ABOUT RHYTHM & FLOW

Giving your speech rhythm is a major key to keeping the audience's attention. Why is it that we remember song words but not dry facts? Why do we have little rhymes to help us remember dates ('In 14 hundred and 92, Columbus sailed the ocean blue'; or the fate of Henry VIII's wives: 'Divorced, beheaded, died; Divorced, beheaded, survived')? Because rhythms appeal to our ears and make speech more attractive.

There's more later about how to change the rhythm with your voice, but here you should be thinking about the rhythm of the actual words themselves. When you're practising your speech out loud, you should be able to hear the beat – if a section feels too clumsy to say, change the rhythm.

There are many ways to introduce rhythm and energy into your speech:

Vary the length of your sentences

I understand. I know abandonment and people being mean to you, and saying you're nothing and nobody, and can never be anything. I understand.

Jesse Jackson, 19 July 1988, taken from *The Penguin Book of Twentieth-Century Speeches.*

Ask rhetorical questions (those you answer yourself)

What, then, are we doing to our capital city now? What have we done to it since the bombing during the war? What are we shortly going to do to one of its most famous areas – Trafalgar Square? Instead of designing an extension to the elegant façade of the National Gallery which complements it and continues the concept of columns and domes, it looks as if we may be presented with a kind of vast municipal fire station, complete with the sort of tower that contains the siren.

Prince Charles, taken from *The Penguin Book of Twentieth-Century Speeches.*

Speak in threes

Our daily deeds as ordinary South Africans must produce an actual South African reality that will reinforce humanity's belief in justice, strengthen its confidence in the nobility of the human soul and sustain all our hopes for a glorious life for all.

Nelson Mandela, 10 May 1994.

Try removing one of the three prongs of Mr Mandela's sentence. The balance goes all wrong, doesn't it? Threes just work.

Echo your phrases

We can never be satisfied as long as the Negro is the victim of the unspeakable horrors of police brutality. We can never be satisfied as long as our bodies, heavy with the fatigue of travel, cannot gain lodging in the motels of the highways and the hotels of the cities. We cannot be satisfied as long as the Negro's basic mobility is from a smaller ghetto to a larger one. We can never be satisfied as long as our children are stripped of their selfhood and robbed of their dignity by signs stating 'for whites only'. We cannot be satisfied as long as a Negro in Mississippi cannot vote and a Negro in New York believes he has nothing for which to vote. No, no, we are not satisfied and we will not be satisfied until 'justice rolls down like waters and righteousness like a mighty stream'.

Martin Luther King.

Use alliteration

What do we want for our children – prison and poverty? Drugs and delinquency? Vandalism and vice? Or peace and positivity? Democracy and dialogue? Victory and valour?

Repeat and reinforce

Repeating words and sounds can help drive your message home.

I know that I will be silenced for many years; I know that the regime will try to suppress the truth by all possible means; I know that there will be a conspiracy to bury me in oblivion.

Fidel Castro, 16 October 1953.

Use imagery and metaphor for added impact

Comparing two things for dramatic effect can be useful. If you have a complicated topic, it can help people understand. Or it can help to paint a mental picture that will inspire the audience. Beware of mixing metaphors (using more than one metaphor at a time).

In his first broadcast as Prime Minister, on 19 May 1940, Winston Churchill knew that Britain was losing the war. Germany was overwhelming every army in its path, but Churchill knew he had to fight on. And he had to get the nation behind him, however hard it might be. Not one for flowery language, he did, however, make use of metaphor in the climax of his speech:

Side by side, unaided except by their kith and kin in the great Dominions and by the wide empires which rest beneath their shield – side by side the British and French peoples have advanced to rescue not only Europe but mankind from the foulest and most soul-destroying tyranny which has ever darkened and stained the pages of history. Behind them –

behind us – behind the Armies and Fleets of Britain and France – gather a group of shattered States and bludgeoned races: the Czechs, the Poles, the Norwegians, the Danes, the Dutch, the Belgians – upon all of whom the long night of barbarism will descend, unbroken even by a star of hope, unless we conquer, as conquer we must; as conquer we shall.

WEB TIP For complete texts of Winston Churchill's speeches, visit **www.winstonchurchill.org**.

Imagery is closely linked to metaphor – and can be equally powerful. Look at these two examples:

Last Tuesday, 8-year-old Johnny Smith was knocked down and seriously injured while crossing the main road through the village.

Or: *Last Tuesday, Mary Smith waved her little son Johnny off to school – just like every mother in this audience. She was just loading the washing-machine when she got the knock at the door that every parent dreads. A policeman had come to tell her that Johnny had been knocked down and was fighting for his life in hospital.*

The first example is perfectly correct, but the second conjures up an emotional image that has an immediate impact on the audience. The first will make them think. But the second will make them feel.

The Reverend Jesse Jackson is a master of language. How many examples of polish can you find in this excerpt from one of his speeches?

I have a message for our youth. I challenge them to put hope in their brains and not dope in their veins.

I told them that like Jesus, I, too, was born in the slum, and just because you're born in a slum does not mean the slum is born in you and you can rise above it if your mind is made up.

I told them in every slum there are two sides. When I see a broken window that's the slummy side. Train some youth to become a glazier; that is the sunny side.

When I see a missing brick, that is the slummy side. Let that child in a union and become a brick mason and build; that is the sunny side.

When I see a missing door, that is the slummy side. Train some youth to become a carpenter, that is the sunny side.

When I see the vulgar words and hieroglyphics of destitution on the walls, that is the slummy side. Train some youth to be a painter and artist, that is the sunny side

We leave this place looking for the sunny side because there's a brighter side somewhere. I am more convinced than ever that we can win. We will vault up the rough side of the mountain. We can win.

GET EMOTIONAL

If your subject is particularly emotional, it's fine to use your feelings to help persuade the audience to your point of view, but let it come naturally. False emotion is all too easily spotted.

TELL 'EM A STORY

Anecdotes can be an extremely useful weapon in your vocal armoury. But irrelevant anecdotes, however amusing they may be, just leave the audience baffled, while they try to work out the link.

CHECKLIST

Make sure your anecdotes do at least one of the following:

Reinforce ❏

Highlight ❏

Explain ❏

Summarize ❏

Tony Blair made history by being the first British Prime Minister to address the Irish Parliament, on 26 November 1998. He made good use of anecdotal material to emphasise the links between himself and the people of Ireland. See how he makes the transition to very personal experiences, without straying from the bigger picture.

Ireland, as you may know, is in my blood. My mother was born in the flat above her grandmother's hardware shop on the main street of Ballyshannon in Donegal. She lived there as a child, started school there and only moved when her father died; her mother remarried and they crossed the water to Glasgow.

We spent virtually every childhood summer holiday up to when the troubles really took hold in Ireland, usually at Rossnowlagh, the Sands House Hotel, I think it was. And we would travel in the beautiful countryside of Donegal. It was there in the seas off the Irish coast that I learned to swim, there that my father took me to my first pub, a remote little house in the country, for a Guinness, a taste I've never forgotten and which is always a pleasure to repeat.

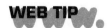

Taken from The History Place, Great Speeches Collection, **www.historyplace.com**.

MAKE 'EM LAUGH

A store detective once told me that the motto of her profession is: 'If in doubt, leave it out.' It's a pretty good motto for many things – jokes in a speech being one of them. Humour is the most difficult thing to get right. And the easiest way of offending people. But everyone likes a laugh and it's a good way to get the audience relaxed, engaged and on your side. So you'll just need to tread carefully.

Try the following sites for some topical gags that you can just throw into your speech:

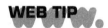

www.bazza.com/sj/humour/

www.jokes-for-all.com

BANISH JARGON

Beware of jargon! You might know what it means, but does your audience? Even if you're talking to a group who should understand the terms, simplify them! Just a slight misunderstanding about a word's meaning can make all the difference.

While we're on the subject of jargon, a quick mention of buzzwords, or management-speak – you know, those phrases that someone always trots out in a meeting. You may work for a company that loves buzzwords, but recent reports have shown most people find them a turn-off.

DON'T ever say:

● Let's run this up the flagpole and see who salutes it.

● Let's put that on the backburner.

● You need to think out of the box.

● Let's touch base.

And don't even think about dreaming up new ones. You'll just sound incomprehensible, like the person who said: 'In order to skin the cat, you need a better mousetrap', or 'I'd like to have a scuba in your think tank' or, perhaps worst of all, 'I want to stick a couple of ideas into your intellectual toaster and see what pops up'.

Think like a listener – not like a speaker.

IDENTIFY YOUR RELATIONSHIP WITH THE AUDIENCE

Put yourself in the audience's shoes and work out what you need to do to keep their attention and help them to remember what you're saying. Visuals, anecdotes and all the stylistic polishes we're talking about in this chapter should help.

DO talk about 'our business', 'our profits', 'the difference we can make', if you're talking to a group that you're part of. Make sure they know that you identify yourself with them.

DO make it clear, if you're not part of the group, that only they can make the difference – motivate them. Talk about 'your rivals', 'your opportunities', 'the best thing you can do'.

DON'T stand up there banging on about 'me' and 'I'.

SUMMARY

Should I write the speech out in full?

Text/script/cue cards. The cue cards will serve you far better.

How should I start?

You need impact, authority and awareness - and make sure it's appropriate.

How do I end?

Pull people together, reinforce your message and demand action. Make sure your ending gives them something to think about.

Polishing your speech

Be chatty, be dynamic, think about rhythm and pace, use imagery and emotion, banish jargon, make 'em laugh and banish jargon.

4

WORDS ARE NOT

ENOUGH

✴ WHY VISUALS ARE IMPORTANT

✴ DIFFERENT TYPES OF VISUAL AIDS

✴ TYPES OF EQUIPMENT

✴ PREPARING YOUR VISUALS

✴ INSIDER TIPS ON WORKING WITH
VISUAL AIDS

✴ USING HANDOUTS EFFECTIVELY

A picture paints a thousand words – and the audience is probably tired of looking at you by now, anyway.

If you've mapped your way through your speech, you'll probably already have had some ideas for visual material. Some points would obviously be better illustrated by a graph or chart of some kind – and you'll already have planned these in.

But you might think about using visuals to emphasise the most important points or to add interest or humour to the presentation. You may even want to think about using sound or video, to add interest or variety, or to explain a point better.

WHY VISUALS ARE IMPORTANT

Pictures are certainly more memorable than words – more even than you might think. A designer who can create a memorable logo for a company is highly prized – and highly paid. The best brands simply seep into your mind, without you even realising. Just seeing that certain shade of pale blue makes me think of Barclay's Bank. And a green carrier bag says Marks & Spencer to me, even if I can't see the company name. Nike's 'swoosh', Coca-Cola's 'dynamic ribbon' and McDonald's 'golden arches' are so instantly recognisable that the manufacturers can use them to brand a product without using the company name at all.

You could simply say: 'Sales figures were rising at a rate of about 2 per cent a year until the introduction of the new system in 1998. Since then, sales have gone up by 25 per cent a year.' But if you show them a graph like this, the information is more likely to stick in their minds.

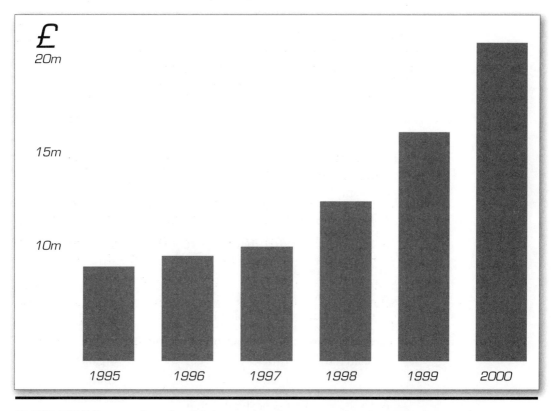

ILLUSTRATION 7:   A graph will help to make information stick in the minds of your audience

CHECKLIST

It's a great idea to include visual material in your presentation, but there's no point in including it if it's not there for a reason.

Go through this checklist and ask yourself: Would my choice of visual material do least one of the following:

show what something looks like?	❏
reinforce a point?	❏
illustrate something abstract or unseen?	❏
show information patterns?	❏
interpret figures?	❏
summarise key points?	❏

Just as logos make a lasting impression so too do visuals used during a speech. They can give a statement real impact and help to explain things like sales figures.

THE RIGHT EQUIPMENT FOR THE RIGHT INFORMATION

Different types of graphics and equipment all have their place, and they're all suitable for different purposes.

- To help the audience remember key points: use key words
- To emphasise easily illustrated specifics: use photographs
- To drive home key points and add humour: use cartoons
- To show something changing over time: use a line graph
- To compare data: use a bar graph
- To show how percentages relate to each other as part of the whole picture: use a pie chart
- To show how departments or events are related to each other: use an organisational chart
- To show a process or step-by-step approach: use a flow chart

- To show key points for large audiences: use slides

- To show key points for a small audience: use an overhead projector (OHP) or a computer presentation

- To show key points for very small audiences or when cash is tight: use a flip chart

- To show an imagined scenario, or to illustrate a narrative point better: use video

Before making a final decision about what visuals you want to use, contact the organisers, or the venue itself, and ask what facilities they have. Some are specially equipped for slides and computer presentations and can project your visual material onto a huge screen, with fantastic quality. It's not going to be a good day if the speaker who's wowing them before you takes advantage of this and then you turn up with your flip chart or handwritten OHP notes that no one beyond row three can even see.

Take some time out of the office – visit the venue to examine the facilities and see how the seating will be set up. Make an appointment to meet the technician there. He or she should be able to give you a demonstration and chat to you about the best approach.

If the venue isn't quite so high-tech, it might still have its own OHP, which would save you taking your own. (See chapter 5 for tips on checking visual equipment.)

>> p. 79
Checking the facilities

If you're using a lot of visual material, you can really make it work for you. Use the visuals as your notes. They'll jog your memory and it'll look impressive if you're not constantly referring to cue cards.

Some experts will try to tell you how many visuals you should include per hour – and this is a useful crutch for people who like to be told what to do. But it is ridiculous to lay down rules about visuals because no two presentations are the same. A presentation about how to identify wild flowers might be based entirely on visuals – imagine how much time you would have to waste in describing those particular colours or petal shapes, without a picture to refer to.

But many of the greatest speeches in the world have conjured up impressive visual imagery, using nothing but the power of words.

However, once you have decided to use visuals it *is* a good idea to present the material fairly regularly throughout your presentation. Let's have a look in more detail at the kinds of visual material that might help back up your points.

DIFFERENT TYPES OF VISUAL AIDS

WORDS Editing your main points down to a few key words is an extremely effective way of driving them home. This form of visual aid is simple, quick and cheap to prepare and can be adapted to tie in with whatever equipment you've decided to use for other support – flip charts, OHPs, computer presentations or slides, for example. It can also look very professional, especially if you use computer-generated graphics.

DO edit ferociously. The key words method will only work if you have no more than about six words.

PHOTOGRAPHS If you work for a design company, for example, or your presentation is deeply rooted in visuals for some other reason, it makes sense to use photographs.

Original photographs can obviously be freely used, although they can take some time to prepare. You may need to gather together the things you want to photograph, or travel to the right place. You will then have to schedule some time to scan them into a computer or allow time for them to be processed as slides.

Or you could invest in a digital camera; they're fairly cheap now. Digital photos can then be downloaded directly into your PC. The advantage of computerised photographs is that you can crop or otherwise alter them with a simple-to-use program such as Photoshop. And when you need them again a year later, the edges won't be all bumped and curled up!

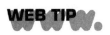

To buy a digital camera, you could visit www.ukdigital cameras.co.uk **or** www.internetcamerasdirect.co.uk **or** www.digital-cameras.com. **If you're not sure what you're looking for, Yahoo!** (www.yahoo.co.uk) **has a particularly useful buyer's guide, as has Computer Shopper** (www.computershopper.com). **Photoshop software can be bought at** www.jungle.com **and other software sites. When I looked, it was priced at about £500.**

If you commission a professional photographer, this can be an expensive exercise. Most photographers charge at least £200 a day for their services, plus the cost of materials. If you have to hire a studio, you're really bumping up the price.

Search for local photographers on Scoot or Yell (the Yellow Pages). You'll find Scoot at www.scoot.co.uk **and Yell at** www.yell.com. **Both sites will allow you to search for services by name, type and location.**

If you use someone else's pictures, you'll probably have to buy them in, paying for the copyright. However, the main photographic agencies are extremely helpful and knowledgeable. You simply call up and describe what you want and they will send you sheets of slides (usually called 'trannies' in the business). There will be a basic search fee and then you pay for the images you use. If you need prints, rather than trannies, professional photographic studios can usually make prints in around 24 hours.

JARGONBUSTER!
Trannies: from 'transparency', i.e. slides.

Many of the main picture agencies have websites, where you can search yourself. Leading photograph agencies include Corbis – **www.corbisimages.com**; Rex Features – 020 7278 87294 – **www.rexfeatures.com**; London Features – 020 7723 4204

DO use photographs for slide and computer presentations as they reproduce well.

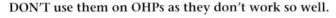

DON'T use them on OHPs as they don't work so well.

CARTOONS These don't have to be hilarious. No one's treating your presentation as a guest spot at the Comedy Store. Unless, of course, it *is* a guest spot at the Comedy Store. In which case, go ahead. Be hilarious.

But even in ordinary speeches or presentations, your audience will probably welcome any attempts at humour if it's appropriate to the subject matter.

DO keep it simple and representational if you decide to draw something yourself. Stick figures will work better than even the best-drawn figures. It's not an art class, it's just meant to get your message across.

If you're using cartoons you've already seen in a publication, remember that copyright laws may apply. Call the publication concerned. They'll usually be able to put you straight in touch with the cartoonist or advise you on the copyright situation.

If you want to commission cartoons, don't forget to include this cost in your budget. To find a cartoonist, you could look at newspapers and publications until you find someone who's doing the kind of work you're after. Trade magazines can be good sources as their resident cartoonist will already know something about your industry. The publication should be able to put you in touch.

WEB TIP

Many cartoonists have their own websites, which enable them to show the range of different styles. For a great directory of links to cartoonists' sites, visit The Cartoonists' Guild's site at www.pipemedia.net/cartoons/index.

GRAPHS AND CHARTS These make all the difference if you're discussing statistics of any kind. Abstract figures can baffle even the most attentive egg-head, but most people can see that a line on a graph which is plunging downwards is news.

TIP

The receptionist at a publication probably won't have a listing for the cartoonist. If the cartoon you like is on the news pages, ask to be put through to the news editor. If it's on a features page, ask for the features editor.

If you're generating your graphs on a computer, you can, of course, come up with all sorts of whiz-bang representations for your charts. These are particularly useful if you're pitching for business and want to impress a client, but simple representations are fine if all you want to do is get your message across. If you, or someone you work with, already know how to do the whiz-bangy things, all well and good. If not, it's easy to get sidetracked into learning how to show company profits as increasingly huge moneybags when you *should* be researching the content of your speech.

Anyway, you should be careful of anything too flashy – sometimes people get carried away with their own cleverness and forget that the purpose of the exercise is to make the statistics easier to read. Too many shadows and logos can get in the way of your message.

DO keep words to a minimum on charts. Make the letters large, clear and plain.

PIE CHARTS If you're using pie charts, make sure the slices tally with the percentages they represent. Use the sofware on your PC to construct the chart and produce a 3-D pie.

By now, you should have a good idea of the best kinds of visual aids to back up your points. But there are so many choices of equipment. Which is the most suitable?

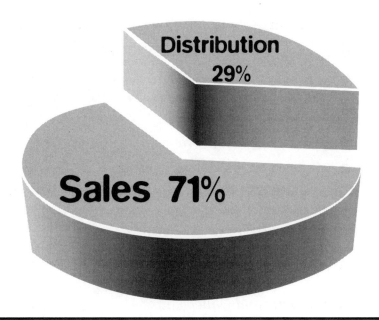

ILLUSTRATION 8:   A pie chart can often illustrate your point better than a graph

TYPES OF EQUIPMENT

Before you decide which type of equipment to use for your presentation, a word of warning: never choose an important speech to use new equipment for the first time. Either use something with which you are familiar, or practise using new gadgets well in advance.

If you need to hire equipment, try visiting www.scoot.co.uk **or** www.yell.co.uk. **If the company has a website, there will usually be a link from Scoot or Yell, so you can simply click through.**

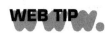

FLIP CHARTS AND WHITEBOARDS

This is the 'back to basics' approach.

DO use a flip chart if:

● you don't have any power for electrical equipment

● you haven't got much money

● you're going to write down audience contributions

● you need to explain things by illustration as you speak

● you've got a small audience

DON'T use one if:

● you really don't want your visuals to look messy

● you're likely to change the running order or refer back (flip charts: it's a pain to flip through all that paper; whiteboards: you might have already rubbed it out)

● you've got illegible handwriting

● you've got a lot to show (size is limited)

With flip charts you can either write the material as you go along, or you can prepare it in advance; using different coloured pens helps to make things stand out and adds variety.

CHECKLIST

Things you'll need for flip charts and whiteboards:

Flip chart

plenty of marker pens in the right colours
   (if you get a dud one, throw it away at
   once so you don't pick it up again) ❑

enough paper in the pad ❑

ruler (if you need one) ❑

something to point with (optional) ❑

Whiteboard

plenty of special whiteboard pens
   (ordinary marker pens are permanent – beware!) ❑

whiteboard rubber ❑

ruler (if you need one) ❑

something to point with (optional) ❑

magnets (if you're using
   other visuals on paper) ❑

You could even get really whizzy and have two flip charts! One, at the left side of the room, could list your main points, while you use the other to go into detail. While you're talking, the audience will be able to remind themselves where they are and what you're talking about.

If you're using a whiteboard, you can also use magnets to secure sheets of paper to the board, which is useful if you want to show other visuals. For whiteboards, 'dry erase' pens are easy to remove, so are better if you want to change things quickly. 'Wet erase' pens are less smudgy and a bit more permanent. But you can still get the marks off with a proper eraser.

DO leave a blank sheet between charts. Sometimes the paper is thin and almost see-through.

DO make a sample chart or sheet and then stand at the back of the room and check that you can see the information clearly. If not, start again. You should check this even if you're planning to write on the sheets as you go along, instead of pre-writing them. It will give you an idea of how big the figures need to be.

DO practise writing quickly and legibly while standing at the side of the board or chart.

DO number the pages if you are pre-preparing a flip chart presentation, so that you don't skip a page and can find your way back if necessary.

DON'T try to write and talk at the same time: you have to turn away from the audience to write and then you won't be able to project your voice properly. Important points may go unheard.

DON'T worry about the silence; the audience will be perfectly happy watching what you're writing. When you've finished writing, turn round and start talking again.

If you're really going back to basics, you could use a blackboard. But that's taking low-tech to almost ridiculous lengths.

TIP

If you are planning to write on the sheets as you go along, you can prepare by lightly pencilling notes in the corners. The audience won't be able to see them and it will look as if you have the memory of an elephant.

PORTFOLIO

A smart folder, possibly with clear pockets on the inside, can be useful. They are used for carrying artwork or other presentation material. Some have a built-in mechanism that allows the portfolio to be propped up, while you flip the sheets over.

 DO use if:

- you're presenting to only a few people

- you're making the same presentation lots of times

- you need the presentation to be very portable

- you can't guarantee you'll have an electrical source

- you need to change the running order, or flip back a lot

- you want to look professional

 DON'T use if:

- you're presenting to a large audience

- you've got more to show than you can fit in the portfolio

 DO buy a strong, good-quality portfolio that's the right size for your presentation material.

DO check that everything is in the portfolio before you go off for a presentation.

DO make sure the light's not glaring off the plastic pockets.

 DON'T use cards or a script for your speech – it will look weird. Use the visuals as your prompt.

OVERHEAD PROJECTORS

An OHP is a lightbox which projects words or images from acetate sheets onto a wall or screen. You can also get a gadget that connects the OHP to your computer, projecting your computer screen onto the wall screen. OHPs have been refined a great deal since the old days. They're now smaller, brighter and project a more even image.

 DO use if:

- you're not very good at technology

- you're worried about equipment breaking down, as they are pretty reliable

- you haven't got much money: they are cheap to buy or hire

- you need to give your presentation in different locations: new models are fairly portable

- you're likely to go back and discuss points you made earlier

- you want to add notes to your visuals as you go along

- you can't darken the room much, as new models are still bright enough to see clearly

DON'T use if:

- it's important that you have a cutting-edge look

- you've got an old model and you're not sure the room will be dark enough and that the machine might be too noisy

- you're worried about damaging or losing the acetates

- you don't have power, a screen or a blank wall

- colours or photographic detail are important to your presentation

Although OHPs don't work well for big audiences, they have the advantage of being flexible. If a question, for example, refers back to one of the visuals, it should be easy to find it and display it once more. With slides, you would have to run through the whole lot. If you can, you should print your OHP sheets on acetate rather than handwriting them. It looks a lot more professional and you can plan out the whole page before you start printing. You can also print an exact copy on paper, for you to refer to, instead of craning your neck round or staring at a brightly lit OHP. You can also hand out the copies after the presentation.

If the presentation includes some pages where you start at the top and work slowly down, remember to exploit the medium. Cover the acetate on the OHP with a piece of paper, which you may then slide down to reveal the points as you speak. This will stop the audience from sneaking a look at what's coming up and thinking about that, instead of what you're talking about now.

Remember to take care of your acetates: put a piece of plain white paper between them as you make them. This will stop them from sticking together. And don't leave them on a hot OHP for too long.

CHECKLIST

Things you'll need for overhead projectors:

Power supply and extension lead, if necessary ❏

Tape to secure the lead to the floor, if it's plugged in anywhere that people might walk. (The best is 'gaffer' tape, or Elephant Tape, available from DIY stores, but any parcel tape will do, as long as it will come unstuck again afterwards) ❏

Screen or wall space ❏

Table with enough room for acetates and your PC (if using it) ❏

Spare OHP bulb ❏

Handkerchief (in case you need to change a hot bulb) ❏

Something to point with (optional) ❏

Acetate marker pens (if you're writing as you go along) ❏

Soft cloth to polish lens and mirror ❏

Once you have placed each sheet on the OHP, stand next to the screen, so the audience doesn't have to gaze at only one or the other. Do this unless you're making notes on the acetate as you go along. If you do make notes, make sure you're not blocking anyone's view. You will find it easier if you place the OHP in the middle of the table. Put the unseen sheets on one side and, as you remove them from the machine, place them on the other side. And finally, try to plan your speech so you don't have to keep switching the OHP on and off – it could blow the bulb.

DO set up before anyone arrives, making sure the image is large enough and not distorted.

DO practise changing the sheets, so that you don't fumble.

DO have a 'title-page' up as the audience comes in. It will look

professional and the audience is less likely to notice the noise of the machine than if you switch it on after they've settled down.

DO check the conditions at the same time you're planning to do the presentation. A new model means the room doesn't have to be very dark. It might be dark enough at 5 pm, but if your presentation is from 9 am to 10 am, the bright morning light could make your visuals invisible.

DO number the sheets, in case you drop the lot on the floor. You might want to mount the acetates in a cardboard frame. They will be easier to handle but bulkier.

DO make sure the actual machine isn't blocking anyone's view.

Use an overhead projector with two bulbs, in case one blows.

SLIDE PROJECTOR

A slide projector is a familiar piece of kit that is now usually powered by remote control and can be linked up with a specially recorded soundtrack, which triggers the slides at the right point in the commentary. They're also a bit brighter and clearer now.

DO use if:

● you can project the image large enough for the room size

● photographic images are important to your presentation

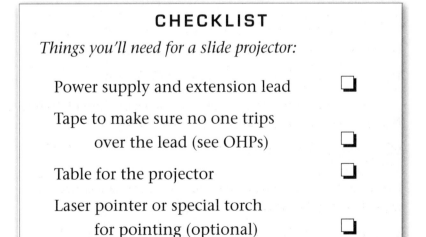

CHECKLIST

Things you'll need for a slide projector:

Power supply and extension lead	❏
Tape to make sure no one trips over the lead (see OHPs)	❏
Table for the projector	❏
Laser pointer or special torch for pointing (optional)	❏

- you need to take your own presentation equipment to the venue (projectors are pretty portable and slides are light and robust)

- you often present using a range of images (slides are easy to get and easy to store)

DON'T use if

- it's important not to put a subconscious barrier between yourself and your audience (turning out the light can do this)

- you don't have power and you can't darken the room at all (although new models are much brighter)

- you might need to change the running order

- you're on a tight budget and you're only going to use the slides once

- you're on a tight deadline and can't wait for the trannies to be produced

When you are preparing your slides, make a mark in the top right-hand corner of the slides, so you don't put them in upside down. Allow time to do a run-through with the projector at the venue before anyone gets there, to make sure the slides are all there and all in the right order.

Remember, if you need to talk about something else between slides, insert a black slide, and if you are using an OHP remove the sheet so that the audience concentrates on what you're saying.

DO number your slides, in case you drop the lot on the floor.

DO use a remote changer and stand by the screen.

DO take a directional lamp or do your speech without referring to notes if you're working in a darkened room.

VIDEOTAPE AND AUDIO TAPE

A change of voice is usually welcomed by the audience and calls them back if their minds were wandering. Copyright considerations might apply, but if you're recording your own footage this will, of course, be fine.

DO use if:

- you want to record delegates acting out scenarios and play them back for analysis

- you need a narrative technique to illustrate your point

- you have a power supply

- you have a big enough TV and/or speakers that are loud enough without distorting

- the venue has a number of TVs linked up to a single video player

DON'T use if:

- (for video) everyone can't see the screen, because of the lighting or the size of the room

DO test the equipment in the room in which you're going to use it.

DO have the tape cued up and ready to go.

DO plan what you're going to do while it's playing. For audio you can stay where you are, for video you should probably sit with the audience and watch it. Try to look interested, no matter how many times you've seen it before.

CHECKLIST

Things you'll need for videotape and audio tape:

Power point and extension lead ☐

Tape for wayward leads (see OHPs) ☐

Video or audio tape ☐

COMPUTER-GENERATED PRESENTATIONS

There are several software packages aimed specifically at presentation, but the best known is Microsoft PowerPoint. No matter which one you choose, they all have the advantage of providing a series of templates. You just fill in the details and – hey presto! – professional graphics. They also give you the option of printing out the pages, so you can easily produce handouts for the audience.

It is also easy for you to store the presentation and alter it later for subsequent presentations. This is useful if you're presenting similar material to different audiences, because you'll be able to tweak the material and personalise it. You can incorporate photographs or video clips into the presentation, which will save you from having to switch equipment part-way through. And you can download images from the internet, or have people mail images direct to your computer.

If you've just learned how to use the software, avoid getting carried away with your new skills. Too many animations and flashing logos can just be distracting.

These are the main options for a computer generated presentation:

1 LCD (Liquid Crystal Display) projection panels – link to an OHP, to project what would normally be seen on a computer screen. The computer can deliver sound at the same time.

2 LCD and DLP (Digital Light Processing) projectors – project the computer screen images onto a wall or screen and deliver stereo sound. Brighter than LCD panels. Many conference centres have systems installed.

3 Large screen computers – suitable for small groups. Speakers provide sound.

DO use if:

● you've got a fast computer with a big memory (when you buy presentation equipment, check with the supplier that your computer will be compatible and fast enough)

● it's important that you appear to be using 'cutting edge' technology

● you make presentations on a regular basis

● you've got some cash to invest in the right equipment

● you're pitching for business and you're in competition with another firm

● your presentations might change at short notice

● the venue has compatible projection equipment, then you'll only need to take a laptop

● the room can't be darkened: most screens work in normal light

DON'T use if:

● you have no idea how to fix it if it goes wrong

● you can't give any kind of presentation if it goes wrong (they can be a bit unreliable)

● you're not sure your PC will be compatible with the projection equipment

● you don't have access to a projector and you're presenting to a large group of people – they'll never all be able to crowd round the screen

● you're hard up

● photographic detail is really important – they're still not quite as good as slide projectors

If you decide to go down this route you should probably go on a course and then practise a lot. Know the hardware and software inside out; it can be very embarrassing if the whole thing goes down at the beginning of the presentation.

DO practise setting up.

DO back up your presentation onto disk and if visual aids are vital, put an OHP or slide projector (plus accessories) in the car, just in case. Or take an expert with you.

DO link to the internet in advance if you need to, and then store the information on file, just in case the link doesn't work.

INTERNET, CD AND DVD PRESENTATIONS

If you regularly repeat the same presentation, it might be a waste of time for you to traipse up and down the country yourself. Instead, you might want to put all the information onto the internet or a CD or DVD (Digital Video/Versatile Disk). Your target can watch it whenever they want, can choose which bits they want to look at first (by clicking on the right sections) and can watch it over and over again. They can also pass it on to colleagues or friends.

To get the best out of a CD, internet or DVD presentation, you may want to hire a specialist company.

JARGONBUSTER!
DVD: Digital Video Disk or Digital Versatile Disk. A new generation of information storage. Holds more information than CDs. Extremely high picture and sound quality.

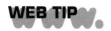

WEB TIP If you're not sure where to find an internet presentation specialist, try typing 'internet presentations' into one of the search engines. In October 2000 there were 1,660 listings, so you shouldn't be short of people to try.

If you're planning to use any kind of visual aid which involves darkening the room, don't schedule it for straight after lunch – everyone will be nodding off. Try to use anything like this in the morning, when everyone is (theoretically) alert. Another disadvantage of darkening the room is that it breaks your eye contact with the audience, so you can't 'read' their feelings about how the presentation is going and rectify any problems.

Once you've thought about what you'd *like* to use, and you've examined what you *can* use, it's time to start preparing your visuals.

TIP

Putting the name and the date of the presentation at the bottom of each page will make the audience think you've done all that work especially for them. Even if you just changed the name and the date from the presentation you did last week.

PREPARING YOUR VISUALS

It is much better to prepare your visuals on a computer. We'll look later at the sophisticated software specially designed for presentations but, that aside, ordinary word-processing packages alone will make all the difference to your visuals. They allow you so much flexibility – you can go back and alter anything at any time.

They also look more professional.

They will allow you to establish a coherent style and design.

WHAT'S YOUR STYLE?

The overall style is the first thing to consider when preparing visual material. Firstly, choose a font by clicking on the Format button on your computer tool bar. Play around with the fonts on your computer, but don't get carried away!

Apart from the style of the lettering, you should also decide on the size, colour, where you put the words on the page and whether you're going to use boxes, borders, symbols or bullet points, etc. Think about the overall design and the presentation will hang together as a coherent whole.

If you're not sure of your way around your word-processing program, it's worth buying a book. Don't be scared of going to a computer store to buy a guide; they're not all full of geeks who'll laugh if you don't *some fonts are fiddly and difficult to read*

OR JUST TOO SQUASHED UP

or simply trying too hard

But some are friendly and clear

Some can look like notes. This might be useful

Some can look old-fashioned.

Don't use them if you're talking about a product that's supposed to be state of the art.

ILLUSTRATION 9:   Different fonts can determine the style of your presentation know what you're talking about. If you're not convinced, go to **www.amazon.co.uk** and use the search tools to find the book you want.

JARGONBUSTER!

Point size refers to the size of letters on a computer.

Make sure you choose a 'point size' that can be seen at the back of the room. It can be changed in the Format menu on the toolbar at the top of the screen or by going to View on the same toolbar, scrolling down to Toolbars and selecting Formatting. Then you'll be able to change the point size as you go along, without going into Format all the time. Simply click on the arrow and scroll down to the number you want.

Be consistent about where you use italics, underlining, bold or centred text, etc.

Think about what colours to use. Dark colours show up better than light ones. Even red can fade away in the wrong light. But try to use different colours for variety, and use them consistently. You might want to assign a certain colour to a certain issue, name or subject.

And don't forget that we associate different colours with different emotions or subjects. Here are a few examples:

RED = stop, danger or hot

GREEN = go, safe, natural, calm, neutral

BLUE = water, cool, efficient, corporate

PURPLE = wealth, luxury, wackiness

YELLOW = sunlight, warmth

Try writing 'GO!' in red or 'HOT!' in green. Some people don't find this particularly freaky, while others find it very weird, so bear it in mind when deciding on colours. Also remember that however warm and sunny it might be, yellow barely shows up at all against white.

Avoid sloppy spelling, poor punctuation and grammatical gremlins.

Your words are going to be on display to everyone – possibly on a massive screen above the stage. Now is not the time for sloppy and inconsistent spelling and shaky grammar.

MAKE SOME RULES FOR YOURSELF!
Make yourself a style-guide: a list of words and punctuation to look out for, including correct spelling and whether a word has a capital letter at the beginning – and stick to it.

CAPITAL LETTERS Many people fall into the trap of scattering capital letters around like they're going out of fashion, especially if they're giving a presentation. Maybe they think it makes the words look more important. Capital letters are for the beginnings of sentences and for proper nouns, such as London Road, Jacey Lamerton and Essential Books.

I've broken my own rules a couple of times in this book – for example by giving capital letters to Objective and End Result. This is because I'm turning them into proper nouns for the purposes of the book and I want them to stand out. You might want to start your bullet points with capital letters. It's up to you. But make it consistent.

DATES AND TIMES Decide how you're going to write these and stick to your rule.

Most English newspapers write 'day, date, month, year' – Thursday 23 March 2000 (note that the date number stands alone, so it's 1 April, 20 May – not 1st April, 20th May).

You may also write times as 5 pm or 17.00 hrs – you decide. No system is *right*; just choose the one you feel comfortable with and stick to it.

QUOTATIONS If you're using quotations, decide how you're going to identify them. Here are a few suggestions, pick one (or make up your own):

'The future doesn't belong to the fainthearted.'

Ronald Reagan, 28 January 1986

'The future doesn't belong to the fainthearted.'

Ronald Reagan, *28 January 1986*

'The future doesn't belong to the fainthearted.'

RONALD REAGAN, 28 January 1986

'THE FUTURE DOESN'T BELONG TO THE FAINTHEARTED.'

Ronald Reagan, *28 January 1986*

ACRONYMS It's clearer and more modern NOT to put full stops in acronyms, e.g. UNESCO. This also applies to people's names, e.g. James T Kirk.

SINGULARS In the written word, companies are singular. Yes, it sounds weird when you say it out loud but it's correct. So you should say: 'Granada Television makes programmes.' The singular rule also applies to:

Team (unless you're writing for the sports pages, in which case it's plural – don't ask me why there's one rule for the front of the paper and another for the back, it's just one of those journalistic anomalies)

Staff

Government

Department

Group

Committee

APOSTROPHES Probably the grammar point most likely to trip people up.

These are the most common problem words:

It's = It is

Its = The thing belonging to it – *The car was new but its tyres seemed worn*

You're = You are

Your = When something belongs to you – *Your dog has fleas*

There's = There is

Theirs = Something belonging to them – *That car? Oh, it's theirs.*

The dog's bowl = The bowl belonging to the dog. One dog.

The dogs' bowl = The bowl belonging to the dogs. One bowl. More than one dog.

The cat's whiskers = The whiskers belonging to the cat. One cat. Lots of whiskers.

If ONE person owns the book, the apostrophe goes BEFORE the 's'.

If MORE THAN ONE person owns the book, the apostrophe goes AFTER the 's'. It doesn't matter how many books there are. That's irrelevant.

CHECKLIST

Are my visuals:

legible? ❑

full of the right amount of information? ❑

the right size so even those at the back can see? ❑

in the right font? ❑

in a consistent style? ❑

checked for spelling? ❑

checked for grammar? ❑

double-checked for figures? ❑

If your word processor has a grammar check it will underline problem words or phrases in green. Take note: 99.9 per cent of times, you'll be right and the computer will be wrong. But just check those bits over again.

If your grammar is not too hot, mug up with one of the latest guides – they're not as dull as they used to be! Good ones to try include *Mind the Stop* by G V Carey, published by Penguin, or the *Oxford Dictionary for Writers and Editors*. Or you could try Strunk & White: *The Elements of Style* at www.columbia. edu/acis/bartleby/strunk.

TIP

Grammar not too hot? Ask at your local library for one of the modern grammar guides.

INSIDER TIPS ON WORKING WITH VISUAL AIDS

The more fancy-schmancy the equipment, the more chance there is that it could go wrong. So think carefully about what you are going to use and make sure you have a backup in reserve if possible.

DO remove any visuals left behind by the previous speaker – you don't want the audience's minds lingering on what someone else has told them.

DO look at the audience, not your visual aids.

DO check, check and double-check the figures you use for any charts or graphs.

DO stand on the left of the screen, from the audience's point of view. They will read from left to right and it will make more sense to them if you're on the left.

DO make sure you know where everything is if you need to dim the lights.

DO allow yourself plenty of time to get familiar with the equipment.

DO structure your speech so that the visual aids support your most important points.

DON'T use visuals that people can't see – if you see what I mean.

USING HANDOUTS EFFECTIVELY

Of course it wouldn't happen to you, would it? You do all this work; you plan your speech meticulously; you write it lovingly, packing it full of all the best and most dynamic words you can summon up; you illustrate it thoughtfully; you deliver it clearly and rousingly; and you answer questions knowledgeably and graciously. And then the audience walks out of the room and forgets every damn thing you've just said. No. It would never happen to you.

But just in case pigs start to fly or Hell freezes over – or maybe just in case human beings act like human beings and have flawed memories, you'd better think about handouts.

WHAT SHALL I GIVE THEM?
Handouts for every presentation will vary but, depending what you're speaking about, you might want to provide:

1 a timetable, especially for a conference, or presentation lasting several hours or days

2 a list of your key points

3 copies of your visual aids

4 information about you

5 a list of sources or further reading suggestions

6 a proposal

And remember to continue the style and grammar structure you worked out for your visual aids.

Even if you're told how many people will be in the audience, check numbers the day before the presentation. You don't want to waste resources by printing off dozens of copies when only six people are going to attend. Having said that, when you've confirmed numbers, chuck in a couple of spare copies, just in case.

PITCHES

If your speech is a professional pitch for business, you'll probably have a proposal anyway. The client will obviously receive a copy of that.

SHOULD I JUST GIVE THEM SOME BITS OF PAPER?

Handouts printed on to A4 and stapled together are perfectly acceptable. However, if you really want to make a good impression, and you've got a bit of a budget, you might want to invest in some kind of wallet or folder.

The simplest ones may just be acetate folders, or you might have access to a binder or laminator. Always print a title-page and use a colour printer, if you have access to one.

Always include your own contact information. If you do a good job, audience members might hire you in the future, or pass on your name to friends and colleagues.

Even if you make presentations regularly, it's highly unlikely that you will be making *exactly* the same presentation over and over again. So it's probably not worth having your handouts printed into a booklet.

Because corporate brochures are so quickly out of date, invest in professionally designed folders, which include pockets for loose-leaf sheets. These can then be printed in large numbers (saving money on print costs) and used by all the different departments – they simply insert their own sheets into the folder.

You might also want to include a specially cut slot in your folder to hold a business card.

ANYTHING ELSE?

You may want to offer them a transcript of your presentation. If your speech is fairly rigid and prepared, you might want to take a few copies along with you. If lots of people want a copy and you don't have enough, offer to forward it to them. If you're speaking more spontaneously, you could record the speech and then prepare a transcript, which can be posted to anyone who requests it.

WHEN SHOULD I HAND THINGS OUT?

If your presentation has a clear timetable, it's best to hand this out before the speech. If the audience know where they are, it will stop them wondering how long they've got to wait until a tea-break.

Knowing there's going to be a change of any kind can also act as a subconscious wake-up call. You can leave this material on their seats, ask someone to hand it out as the audience enters or, if you're addressing a small group, it's more friendly to hand it out personally.

Biographical material about you is also better handed out before. It could be posted out in advance, although some people will inevitably not read it. If you hand it out immediately before the session starts, it might distract people. The best time might be as people arrive, particularly if you're serving tea or coffee first.

Reading the information will give people something to do while they wait for the speech to start. If the members of the audience don't know each other, it might also help to break the ice.

The printouts of your visual aids, however, are a different question. My advice would be to hand them out in advance only if really necessary. Any material given out in advance can be a distraction. Don't do anything that might drag them away from your words of wisdom!

When presenting your first visual aid, let people know you will be handing out copies of all visual material at the end of the session. That way, they won't be anxiously trying to copy your graphs and charts and they can sit back and concentrate on what you're saying.

BUT THEY'RE STAYING FOR COFFEE AFTER THE SESSION – WON'T THEY LOSE THE NOTES?

Now you're getting cynical! You're probably right, though. The best time to hand out your support material is when your audience is about to leave the venue – whether that's immediately after your speech or a while later.

You might want to give people the option of posting the notes to their offices. Or, if you know the names of all the delegates in advance, you might want to produce personalised notes.

Not only will they feel more obliged to take care of them, you'll be able to forward them if they *do* get left behind.

COPYRIGHT

Copyright can be a tricky area, which you're most likely to encounter when preparing visual aids. It can refer to text, letters, art, audio, advertisements, maps, charts and tables – even to information published on the internet, so beware! This doesn't mean you can't use copyright material – but you need to check what credit you should give and if you need to pay a fee.

Photographs are also copyright – and the photographer owns the copyright, unless it was taken during the photographer's employment, in which case it belongs to the employer. If you commission photographs, it doesn't mean you hold the copyright, unless this was arranged in a written agreement.

The same rule applies to all material – if it's created in employment, or signed over, it belongs to the employer or commissioner. If not, it belongs to the originator.

Photocopying can, surprisingly, infringe two sets of copyright: that of the creator of the work, *plus* that of the publisher, who has typeset the page.

If you're presenting copyright material for the purposes of reviewing it, you don't normally need to get formal permission – as long as credit is given. This means written acknowledgement of the author and publication alongside the material you have used. If you're not sure who to credit, get in touch with the publisher (see below).

If you're presenting to the public or any event for which people have paid, you'll need to get proper permission to show copyright material, and you might have to pay a fee. Again, you should contact the publisher.

You can use extracts from magazines or books in your presentations, but beware, because the law is very hazy on this point. Reproducing a

JARGONBUSTER!
Copyright: the sole legal right to print, publish or perform film, or record a literary, artistic or musical work.

'substantial amount' needs permission, but no one really knows what this means!

To try to help, some bodies have set down clearer guidelines, known as 'fair dealing', about how many words you can reproduce without permission. BUT these guidelines only apply to material used for criticism or review and you will need to include the author's name and the title of the book (it's also courtesy to include the publisher's details).

But bear in mind that these guidelines are not included in law and they don't cover music, lyrics, work to be used in anthologies, work which has been changed in any way, or complete articles, however short.

It's always best to check with the copyright holder before going ahead.

When you write to the publisher, or other copyright holder, you need to:

- ask for non-exclusive permission to reproduce the item
- include details of where you'll be reproducing it from
- include an explanation of what you want to use it for
- ask exactly what credit you need to publish
- ask if your planned acknowledgements are OK

The fair dealing guidelines say you can reproduce:

400 words as a single extract, from a single book

800 words as various extracts from a single book, provided no individual extract is more than 300 words

less than a quarter of an article from a newspaper or magazine

less than a quarter of a poem, or a number of extracts that add up to less than a quarter of a poem

For more about copyright issues, try the Copyright Licensing Agency's website, www.cla.co.uk. The site includes details about general copyright issues, up-to-date information about rights concerning the internet, plus links to other bodies dealing with copyright.

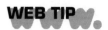

SUMMARY

You now have a good idea of your options with visual aids – you're aware of what to use and when. Let's recap:

Visuals aren't just eye candy

Make sure visual aids are there for a reason.

The right gear for the right fact

Decide which equipment is best at conveying your point.

Preparing your visuals

Establish style and avoid mistakes.

Insider tips

Remember the advice on page 71

Handouts

Give them something they can use – at the right time.

Beware of copyright issues.

5

THE VENUE

✳ CHECKING THE FACILITIES

✳ ADAPTING THE VENUE

✳ SPOTTING POTENTIAL PROBLEMS

When people are asked to speak at an event, the speech takes over every waking thought. But many of the opportunities and potential pitfalls come from the venue itself, and from other presentation techniques, such as the equipment you use to back up your speech. Don't skip this section – I know you're worried about drying up and forgetting your words but this is really where most things go wrong!

If you've booked the venue yourself, you'll need to be even more careful. Don't worry about upsetting the caretaker – make sure they know EXACTLY what you need and make sure you have all their contact details in case there's a problem. Get the details of the booking in writing.

Make sure the audience have the correct information, too.

Of course, you already know what the venue looks like, don't you? Because you're Mr/Ms Organised, aren't you? You checked it out and discussed the facilities before you even set pen to paper, didn't you? You'll already have requested a mike and PA system, plus spares for the audience to use during question and answer sessions.

You'll have told them you need a flip chart and an OHP and you'll have discussed where that should be. Then you called the day before, to double-check they knew what your requirements were.

TIP

It might sound obvious but double-check the time, date and venue of the presentation and call the day before to check everything's still on course.

CHECKING THE FACILITIES

Now you've arrived at the venue in plenty of time and you're going to check that everything's in order.

If, because of distance or some other reason, you can't visit the venue beforehand, get the name of the facilities manager or caretaker and have a detailed chat about the venue.

Remember – it's a pain, but getting there in plenty of time could mean hours before you're actually 'on'. You might not be speaking at the conference until 12 noon, but if the first speaker starts at 9 am, you'll need to get there around 8 am to check that everything's working. If it's not, that will give the facilities people time to do something about it. Don't worry – you can while away the intervening time by criticising other people's speaking techniques!

If you're not speaking at a venue that's accustomed to hosting presentations, you'll have to do a bit more work yourself.

Arm yourself with a mental straggly beard and long greasy hair, because we're heading into Roadie territory.

Certain elementary checks may seem too basic to bother with but the simplest of things can go wrong and scupper your presentation.

POWER POINTS AND EXTENSION LEADS

In a conference venue, these should be plentiful and well placed. If you're speaking in the church hall, though, you might find the points are all at the 'wrong' end of the room.

Even if you do see a point in the right place, don't assume that it's working: check it!

Work out how many power points you need and where they need to be. If there aren't enough in the right place, make sure you take a four-plug extension lead to the presentation.

ELECTRICAL EQUIPMENT

We looked at electrical equipment in the last section, so you should be fairly clear about the choices, advantages and possible pitfalls.

But don't forget:

DO test the equipment beforehand – at the venue.

DO take a simple repair kit of spare bulbs, electrical screwdriver, masking tape, scissors and fuses; or,

DO take a flip chart or other low-tech alternative in case the whole thing goes wrong. If a piece of equipment is vital to your presentation, get the number of an engineer who offers an express service.

SOUND EQUIPMENT

TIP

A top showbiz tip is to position the mike about half an inch below your chin: you'll be less likely to get feedback from being too close to it and the audience will be able to see your face. Bonus!

Get someone to help you do a sound check. The best way to test the mike is by speaking into it. It's easy to get overenthusiastic when you're tapping it and you'll either deafen the audience or break the equipment.

HEALTH AND SAFETY

While you're still planning which electrical equipment you'd like to use, it's worth bearing a few health and safety rules in mind. If you've got a crowd of people tramping in and out, *one* of them is bound to trip over that trailing lead that you thought would be OK. And if that person is you, that's even more embarrassing.

If you *must* have cables trailing across the floor, make sure they're taped down securely. The best tape to use for this is the 'gaffer' tape or 'elephant' tape used by television crews. It's usually black or grey and about two inches wide. You can buy it from DIY stores but most venues will have a supply. Ask in advance!

TOILETS AND FIRE EXITS

If the audience is unfamiliar with the venue, they will need to be told where the toilets and fire exits can be found. You might want to make these kind of 'housekeeping' announcements, including when they can expect a cup of tea, before you start your presentation proper.

If there is an emergency, don't forget that they'll think of you as being in charge. If an alarm goes off, don't dither about, thinking it might be a drill. Tell people calmly and clearly to make their way to the fire escape (remind them where it is) and to assemble at the fire assembly point (remind them where that is, too). If it turns out to be a false alarm, shepherd them back in again and make sure everyone's settled before you re-start.

And don't be put off your stride – emergencies tend to break down barriers and the audience will probably be far more jovial than they were before.

REFRESHMENT ARRANGEMENTS

Make sure you know what time you're due to break for coffee/lunch/the end of the day, so that you can pace yourself.

If refreshments are to be served in the same room, try to arrange for the caterers to wait outside until you tell them you're ready. Otherwise you might have got to the very climax of your speech, only to have the wind taken out of your sails by a doughty tea-lady, clattering her steel teapot against the plate of custard creams.

If you're in charge, make sure there's somewhere to make and serve the refreshments you have in mind. You'll need a kitchen with the right equipment, crockery, cutlery, a serving table, napkins, and possibly staff to make it, serve it, clear up and wash up.

If you want to offer a glass of wine, say, after the presentation, check first with the management. Many church halls don't allow alcohol to be consumed on the premises. The same goes for smoking. Make sure you tell people if they have to go outside to smoke – and ask them to be considerate about what they do with ash and cigarette ends.

While tea-breaks revive, lunch can send people to sleep. Try to wriggle out of doing your presentation immediately after lunch.

If you're talking all day, or if you *have* to have the post-lunch slot, bear that in mind when you're planning your presentation. Don't give them the most vital bits of info while they're nodding off under the weight of the steamed pudding they never normally eat but to which they've just treated themselves. Not to mention the delights of the bar to which a few always sneak off.

TIP

Don't present vital information to a dozy lunchtime audience.

ADAPTING THE VENUE

SEATING

You might not be able to change this but, if you can, it's worth thinking about the best seating configuration for your needs.

Think about what you want to achieve.

A lively discussion, with lots of input from the audience?

Seat them in a U-shape. If it's a small meeting, seat them around a central table. If there are more people, arrange the tables and chairs in the U-shape. If you want it to be very lively and informal, don't give them tables at all.

Hold their attention – they can talk about it later.

Seat them in rows, facing you. They might still whisper to their neighbour, but they'll be less likely to make eyes at the person opposite – or flick elastic bands at them.

OTHER FURNITURE

DO make sure there's a table for an overhead projector or handouts for people to take as they leave the room.

DO make sure there's somewhere to set cups if people are going to have tea and coffee during the presentation.

DO give them something to lean on if you're going to ask them to take lots of notes.

SIZE

If you're in a huge barn of a room, with half a dozen people, it can make the presentation feel cold and flat, while the audience feels uncomfortable. If you can, move the furniture to make the room cosier. Ask if there are any room-dividers, display boards, large plants or anything that can be used to make the space more intimate.

If it's going to be too small, there's not much you can do except move to a completely different, larger venue, or just put up with it.

LIGHT AND SHADE

Make sure the lighting's appropriate and that you're not either blinded or standing in a dark corner, where the audience can barely see you. Equally, if you have visuals, you might need the lights down for a slide presentation. Make sure your visuals aren't ruined by glaring sunlight through a window that has no blinds.

DO tape up some black card at the windows if there are no blinds or curtains. It's not ideal, but if your visuals are very important to the presentation, the audience will have to see them.

DO rehearse closing and opening blinds or curtains that are there. You'll feel a fool if you're bumbling about with your back to the audience.

ATMOSPHERE

This is a tricky one to put your finger on, but can make or break your presentation. If the room is shabby but there's nothing you can do about it, you might want to take some display boards and pin up information about your company or campaign. If the place is a bit 'dead' and flat, a tablecloth, vase of flowers or plants might make all the difference. If you're at a hotel, ask the manager if they can supply these. Or pack your own.

If you're doing a business presentation, shabby and mismatched furniture could present the wrong impression. Consider hiring furniture for the occasion – it's not as expensive as you might think.

Find a local furniture hire company through Scoot or Yell (www.scoot.co.uk **and** www.yell.com). **Or you might want to get to know a company that offers a nationwide service. Try** www.roomservicegroup.com **or** www.denbe.com.

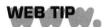

HEATING AND VENTILATION

Ideally, you should be able to change this within the room itself. If not, find out who can put the heating on if things get too chilly. Check if you can open a window if it gets too hot, but think about fans if the window opens on to a busy road, a school playground, or if you're in an airport flightpath. (See below for advice on how to deal with noise, and other distractions.)

You need your audience to be comfortable – too hot and they'll nod off through even the most thrilling presentation; too cold and they'll find it equally hard to concentrate and they'll be uncomfortable if they're muffled up in gloves and coats, dreaming about the hot cuppa they might get at 11 am.

SPOTTING POTENTIAL PROBLEMS

While you're still in Roadie mode, apply your new-found venue expertise to spotting possible distractions. Some of these you won't be able to do anything about, such as fire alarms going off or emergency vehicles screaming past, in which case you need to know how to handle them.

Others, you can do something about; but only if you recognise them as potential distractions. Here are some scenarios and possible solutions:

1 The venue is near a busy road which creates a great deal of background noise when the windows are open, but it's hot and we need air.

DO get there early and open all the windows as wide as possible, to get some air circulating.

DO close the window when you're ready to start; the sudden reduction in noise should actually help get the audience to quieten down too.

DO open the windows during any breaks. Request fans if it's really very hot.

DON'T open the windows if it is very noisy. Request or hire some fans, and specify that you need ones that operate quietly.

2 There is actually air conditioning but it's too noisy and people at the back of the room can hear nothing but the whirring of the machine's fan.

Treat this as you would the busy road (above). Switch off the system while you're talking, cranking it right up during any breaks if possible.

3 There's a loud ticking clock and it will hypnotise the audience to the extent that they'll fall asleep.

When you assess the venue in advance, ask if the clock can be stopped. If not, you'll have to work harder to counter its sleep-inducing effects.

DO move about, ask questions, use visuals etc.

DON'T talk with a clock right behind you. Cover it up or move it. Instead of listening to you, the audience will be grimly fascinated by how slowly its hands are moving.

4 It's a beautiful day and the sun is streaming in. People will be getting too warm and again might start to feel sleepy.

Use the methods above to keep the temperature down. It might be a bit miserable to shut out the sun, but you'll need to do it if it's very bright.

DO allow people to move their seats out of the direct sunlight if there are no blinds or curtains.

DO schedule some extra breaks and, on their return, ask if anyone needs to move.

DO try to be considerate about the environment; some people find that sunlight easily triggers migraine or sickness, not ideal conditions under which to absorb your presentation.

5 The room has a big window with an interesting view, but the view might just be too distracting.

Again, you'll have to be a miseryguts and close the curtains. If this isn't possible, try to change the layout of the room so that the window is behind, or to the side of the audience.

6 There's some sudden, but passing noise such as an emergency vehicle, a low-flying aircraft, a refuse lorry, etc.

DON'T pretend it's not there and simply get louder and louder. Your speech might be important but the rest of the world hasn't stood still.

DO stop and resume once the noise has gone. If you can, say 'I'll just pause while that plane goes over', then make a joke or light-hearted remark if you can, remind the audience what you were discussing and continue.

7 There's a lot of noise from the office outside the room.

If you think this is likely, stick a notice on the door, asking for quiet.

SUMMARY

You now know how important the venue can be. This section is a bit nerdy: there's lots to remember and there's lots to forget. I've put together a detailed checklist – tick it off before you go any further!

ASK YOURSELF:

Have I:

Checked the time, date and venue? ❑

Got the details of the booking in writing? ❑

Booked it on a day the audience can make? ❑

Have I remembered:

My notes! ❑

Any handouts? ❑

Extension leads? ❑

Gaffer tape? ❑

Any presentation equipment not being provided by the venue? ❑

Spare bulbs for OHP or slide projector? ❑

Spare fuses? ❑

Pens etc. for visual aids? ❑

Electrical screwdriver? ❑

Any catering equipment not being provided? ❑

Black card (if there is bright sunlight and no blinds)? ❑

Display boards or room-dividers (if necessary)? ❑

Information about my company or campaign (if appropriate)? ❑

A tablecloth, vase of flowers or plants (if needed)? ❑

A notice asking for quiet (if needed)? ❑

SUMMARY

Have I remembered to check:

Fire exits? ❑

Fire assembly point? ❑

Toilets? ❑

Refreshment arrangements? ❑

Power points? ❑

Sound equipment? ❑

Visual aid equipment? ❑

That trailing leads have been taped down? ❑

Refreshment arrangements? ❑

That I can offer wine (if wanted)? ❑

Smoking regulations? ❑

That the seating is organised as I want it? ❑

That any other necessary furniture is all there? ❑

That any hired furniture is definitely arriving? ❑

That I can close the blinds or curtains? ❑

That any additional 'dressing' for the room is there? ❑

Who can put the heating on/how to work it? ❑

Who can put the air-conditioning on/how to work it? ❑

Whether I can open a window? ❑

That clocks are stopped or unobtrusive? ❑

6

PERSONAL

PRESENTATION

✳ NERVES

✳ YOUR VOICE

✳ WHAT SHOULD I DO WITH MY BODY?

✳ ESTABLISHING CONTACT WITH THE

AUDIENCE

Having spent so much time and energy preparing for your presentation, you may well be worried that you will let yourself down by becoming some kind of nervous wreck or suddenly developing an inability to control your arms and legs.

Don't worry. This chapter will, hopefully, give you some pointers on how to settle your nerves before, or even during, a presentation. You should also be able to use the advice in here to avoid moving or gesturing like a cartoon character.

Without a doubt, if you are able to put into practice even some of the advice laid out here, it should help you to develop enough confidence to tackle any situation, or to maintain your own confidence at a level that allows you to take almost anything in your stride.

NERVES

We've all heard famous and accomplished actors, politicians and television presenters banging on about how it's *good* to feel nervous – that we need a certain amount of extra adrenalin pumping round to make us perform at our best. That's all very well for them. The difference is that they know how to handle it and we ordinary bods simply don't.

So there it is, the nerves will come. The question is, how to stop your mouth going dry, your tongue gumming up, your hands shaking like a jelly and your voice sounding like that of a 90-year-old with a sore throat.

By now, you'll have done all your preparation and the speech has been honed to a veritable work of art. Keep reminding yourself that you've done all the groundwork and that should help a bit.

Emma used to swim competitively as a child. She was so nervous before her first gala that she was sick six times before she even got to the leisure centre. She recalls that standing at the end of the pool, waiting for the starter's gun, was a form of torture. Even now, she says she can't watch swimming races on the television without feeling a shadow of that former terror. But she also remembered: 'As soon as the whistle blew and I was in the water, my nerves disappeared. I was just concentrating on my stroke, my breathing and my strength. I didn't give those nerves another thought.'

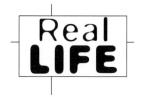

The chances are, the same will happen to you, as soon as you get the first words out of your mouth.

Remember that you're speaking to an audience of ordinary people who have the same fears and hopes as you have.

I'll bet you can talk to your partner or speak up in front of three, five or ten of your closest friends. It doesn't matter if you're speaking to three people or three hundred people. They're all individual people who know that speaking in public can be a bit daunting. You're not making a presentation to three hundred evil geniuses. Unless you're Ming the Merciless, in which case, if they heckle, you can just have them killed.

Other than that, you need to ask yourself a couple of questions.

- What am I afraid of?

- Is the worst likely to happen?

- Is there anything I can do about it if it does?

Now, let's look at a few of the most common fears.

- I might dry up.

- They might listen to me when I'm chatting in the pub but I'll never keep their interest for 30 minutes.

- I'm worried about my accent.

- I'm worried I won't use the right words.

- Someone in the audience might be an expert on this subject.

- Someone might ask a question I can't answer.

- Someone might heckle me.

Thinking about some of the questions above, let's see if those fears are founded, and what you can do about them.

I MIGHT DRY UP!

Yes, you might. Even the most seasoned professional will sometimes grind to an inelegant halt.

So plan what you're going to do if you dry up.

DON'T waffle on, expecting the words to come back to you miraculously – you'll spend all your energy cringing at the rubbish you're talking.

DON'T worry if you can't exactly remember the clever way you were going to convey the point. Just get the message across and the audience will never know they missed out on your best *bons mots*.

DON'T over-apologise.

DO look at your notes – that's what they're there for.

DO give yourself pause for thought to find the right words – it might seem like an eternal silence to you, but the audience will be grateful to you for marshalling your thoughts. It's the adrenalin that's making it feel like ages.

Have a quick look back at chapter 3 where we discussed how much to put in your notes and how much to keep in your head. Make sure you jot down figures and quotes because they are the only things that need to be accurate and the most likely to go clean out of your head!

I'M NO RACONTEUR – WON'T EVERYONE GET BORED?

>> p26

Deciding on the words

If you've researched, mapped, written and polished your speech properly (see chapter 3), there's no reason why they should be bored. You've already thought about rhythm, balance, contrast and visuals. You're not a stand-up comedian and you're not auditioning to be the audience's best friend. You're not Churchill, rallying the nation. You're an ordinary person, speaking in the 21st century. You're there to put across your message in the most effective way.

DO keep your tone fairly conversational and you'll avoid the stilted 'lecture' that does bore people.

I'M WORRIED ABOUT MY ACCENT

Hang-ups about accents are much less common these days, with 'BBC English' risibly historic and our screens and cities populated by a wide cultural and economic mix. Everyone thinks they sound horrible the first time they hear their own voice – it's a cruel twist of nature. Famous speakers don't worry about their voice – they worry about getting their message across.

DON'T try to be something you're not – the accent will slip and you'll really look stupid.

DO think about making yourself understood. As I said before, you're there to put across a message, that's all.

DO think yourself lucky that you'll sound different from the last speaker. The audience will relish the change.

I'M WORRIED I WON'T USE THE RIGHT WORDS

Highly unlikely, if you're familiar with conversational English. Because if you're worrying about long words or jargon, you're better off without them. You may not have the vocabulary of Dr Johnson on the tip of your tongue – but neither will your audience.

DO try to be clear and concise.

DON'T try to impress the two or three audience members who know what your long words actually mean.

WHAT IF THERE'S AN EXPERT IN THE AUDIENCE?

If you've done all the research – YOU'RE an expert now! And if they're such an expert, what are they doing in the audience? Well, I do concede you might encounter a specialist, but don't be so defensive! See the sections on heckling and difficult questions in chapter 7.

>> p114
Dealing with difficult people

DO use them as a resource – someone to add to your ideas.

DON'T forget that you're in charge – you've got the mike, the clock, the platform, the snazzy whiteboard or overhead projector. It doesn't matter how much they know – it's YOU that's been invited to speak and you're doing just that.

SOMEONE MIGHT ASK A QUESTION I CAN'T ANSWER

See chapter 7 for more help with answering difficult questions.

>> p114
Dealing with difficult people

It is true that there is about a 50/50 chance of this happening to you, depending on the topic. However, if you've done all your research, you should have covered all the obvious bases.

DO turn the question back – 'I don't know, I've never thought about that. Why do you ask?'

DO consider whether the question is relevant to your presentation – if not, suggest you discuss it after the speech.

DO promise to find out later and get back to the questioner if you decide it's a valid point.

DON'T worry if you don't know everything – be confident. No one's come to see the all-seeing, all-knowing being.

DON'T waffle or lie. These sins will find you out – you'll be as transparent as a pane of glass!

SOMEONE MIGHT HECKLE ME

Well, they might – especially if you're planning to be controversial.

>> p117
Insults & putdowns

See the separate section on this; learn a few classy put-downs and don't forget you've got the mike. Just be yourself – only a bit louder, more confident, and slower.

You can get through life without practising what to say. You don't clam up when you ask for your bus ticket. And there's no single 'right' way of asking for the bus ticket. You just start speaking and you get your message across. Once you know what you want, public speaking is no different.

I STILL FEEL NERVOUS!

The way to handle nerves and regain control over your voice is to get control of your breathing. Most of the time we don't think about breathing, it's a reflex action. That's why we don't always have much control over it. Practise this breathing exercise:

BREATHING EXERCISE

1 Sit or stand quietly

2 Breathe in through your nose, count slowly to four and then stop

3 Hold your breath for a count of four

4 Release the breath through your mouth, to a count of four.

For the next breath, try to extend the 'breathing-in' count, until you can count up to maybe 16. But take it slowly, over a matter of weeks. Stop if you get dizzy. Practise a few times a day and then do it just before you start your speech. By then you should have much more control over your breathing and your body will have learned that it's time to relax.

Another surefire way to relax is to tense up. That sounds mad, but it's a yoga trick that really works. If you're feeling nervous just before your speech, nip off to the toilet, or somewhere else that's private, and run through the exercises here in boxes.

RELAXATION EXERCISE 1

1 Breathe in and tense the muscles in your shoulders and neck as tight, tight, tight as you can. Pull your shoulders right up to your ears, tense as hard as you can.

2 Relax. Breathe out and as you do so, push your shoulders back and down and then relax totally.

3 Repeat as many times as you want.

RELAXATION EXERCISE 2

1 Screw your face right up into a horrible grimace (this is why it's important to do this exercise somewhere private). Concentrate on screwing up your mouth, your eyes, your nose, your forehead, your whole face.

2 Stretch out your face as much as you can. Pull your mouth right open, open your eyes as wide as they'll go, even flare your nostrils out.

3 Relax.

DEALING WITH A DRY MOUTH, SHAKING HANDS AND OTHER PHYSICAL TICS CAUSED BY NERVES

GABBLING Sit quietly a few minutes before you're due to start. Take long, controlled breaths in through your nose, hold them a second, then breathe out through your mouth. Don't forget that adrenalin speeds you up, so make an effort to slow down.

DRY MOUTH Have a glass of water nearby and don't forget that you *can* take the time to drink from it.

SNIFFING Blow your nose before you get up and keep a clean handkerchief at hand. If you need to use it, take the time. You're in charge!

LOCKJAW If you're so nervous you feel you can't prise your mouth open, nip into the toilets and do a few muscle relaxing exercises.

1 Roll your shoulders forward, up to your ears, back and down. Repeat ten times.

2 Screw up your face tight and then relax. Make sure no one's watching.

3 Drop your jaw as far as it will go, then open your mouth as wide as it will go. Then relax. Do this a few times to remind your mouth that it can move.

SHAKY HANDS We talked in chapter 3 about the advantages that cards have over paper, one of them being that the shaking looks much worse with paper. If you're a shaker, don't hold your notes. Put them down on the desk.

What you do with your hands depends on what resources you have. You may be able to lean on the desk, or hold on to the lectern. As the speech progresses, you might want to nonchalantly put them in your pockets for a while. Just remember, you feel more awkward than you look.

CALLS OF NATURE Don't let nerves make you drink more coffee, tea or cola than you're used to. Nerves will make you want to wee as it is; they'll just make it worse *and* you'll be shaking like a drug-crazed maniac, thanks to all the extra caffeine. If you're at a conference, avoid the temptation to be the life and soul of the hotel bar the night before.

And whatever you do:

DON'T fidget.

DON'T fiddle (if you're a fiddler, take your change and keys etc. out of your pockets beforehand).

DON'T scratch.

DON'T click your biro.

DON'T grip the lectern so tightly that your knuckles go white.

DO smile (not an idiot grin, but at least try to look as if you want to be there and that you're not going to put the audience through an hour of hell).

ALL OF THE ABOVE – AND WORSE!

If you've got it really bad, you could try two real Californian techniques: visualisation and affirmation. If you're *that* nervous, you've got nothing to lose! This honestly works – people have even beaten cancer with it sometimes. So believe in it and it will help. You weren't born with the hang-ups you've got – you learned them. So you can unlearn them. Try doing this before you go to sleep and you'll have the best chance of reprogramming your subconscious. If you start panicking before you are due to speak, replay your visualisation, use those affirmations to stop the negative thoughts. Just don't allow yourself to dwell on the negative.

Visualise yourself happy and confident on the podium, nodding modestly at the audience's rapturous applause. Or striding manfully across the stage, speaking articulately, your words creating powerful images for the audience, who are simultaneously inspired and charmed by you and your speech.

Then affirm this visualisation by replaying it over and over again – telling yourself it *can* be done, and it *will* become true.

Don't think for a moment that drink will help. If you're nervous to begin with, dulling your faculties will give you an extra reason to be afraid. Go in there as sharp as a pin – and head for the bar straight afterwards if you want!

For more ideas on how to control your nerves, visit:

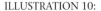 **WEB TIP**

www.stresscure.com/jobstress/speak

college.hmco.com/communication/speech/overcome

For some relaxation exercises, try:

www.easytaichi.co.uk/relaxation_techniques

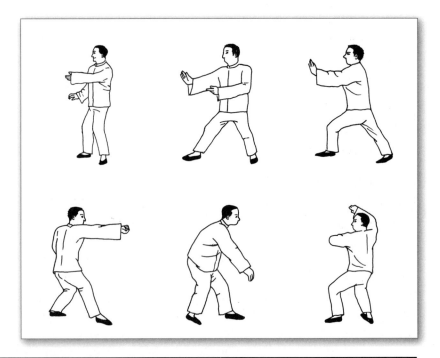

ILLUSTRATION 10:   Tai chi is recognised as an excellent way of relaxing your body

, YOUR VOICE

We've talked at length about the different types of equipment you might want to use as part of your speech, but the most important piece of kit is, of course, your voice. If your voice serves you perfectly well most of the time, it will serve you well in front of an audience, or on radio or television. Voice coaches might tell you an interesting piece of research.

When a voice-trained person delivers information, the audience retains 83 per cent of the content.

When an untrained person delivers the same information, the audience retains only 45 per cent of the content.

Well, I'm not sure about the scientific basis for such research, but I can believe it – up to a point.

Pitch, tone, speed, accent and clarity all help to retain one's interest – and you're more likely to remember something if you've actually listened to it in the first place.

But voice coaches will insist that you need professional training to achieve such results. I don't doubt a professional voice coach *would* improve almost everyone's delivery. But if you're not a regular public speaker, it's probably not worth the time and money.

So let's take the DIY approach for now, and start off by examining the surprising range of factors that have influenced the voice you have. These include:

● the influence of your family, friends and colleagues

● the vocal habits you developed as you grew up

● the physical make-up of your mouth, nasal passages and all the other bits and pieces used in speaking

● your general health

● your personality and outlook

So if any one of those variables changes, it can have an impact on your voice. And you might have to work on one or all of them if you want to change your voice.

I bet that if you've ever heard your voice on tape you'll think it sounds awful. Everyone's voice sounds awful when they're not used to hearing it on tape. The lovely echo chamber that is my head (no jokes please) makes my own voice sound rather resonant and low-pitched to my ears. Vocal glitches and a slight accent sound interesting and possibly even cute.

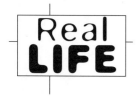

My friend Daisy has to do lots of presentations, as part of her job. When I asked her for her public speaking tips, she let me into a secret and revealed she worries about her accent. She said: 'I'm a bit of a sponge for other people's accents, so I like to think I've developed a "go anywhere" kind of voice – not posh, not common, but universally acceptable.'

But one of her presentations was video recorded and she was horrified by what she heard when the tape was played back. She wailed: 'I sound like some kind of mutant with Sandra Dickinson's high pitch wedded to an accent that veers between the glottal stops and strangled vowels honed by spending my formative years listening to the estuary English of Margate, before escaping to London, working with posh people and living with a Yorkshireman. I've given up listening to tape recordings of my voice. It was giving me anorexia of the larynx.'

Yes, your voice sounds horrible. But only to you. So try not to worry about it.

But if you really do want to change your voice for any reason, be reassured that you *can*. People change their voices all the time. Actors regularly see voice coaches to get the right accent and intonation for a part. People who have had accidents sometimes have to rebuild their voices from scratch.

And, perhaps surprisingly, one of the biggest areas of voice therapy is for transsexuals. The hormones administered during the sex-change procedures do some of the work but the patient usually needs to refine his or her new voice with a course of speech therapy.

So, you *can* change your voice – and if you don't want to change it, you can also make the very best of the voice you have, making it more powerful and resonant.

It takes practice and it takes some time. Get into the habit of practising while you're doing something else – don't sing in the bath, speak! Talk to yourself whenever there's no one around. You'd better tell your partner what you're up to though, or you could find yourself practising in a padded cell. And the acoustics in those places are terrible.

BECOME A LISTENER

Before you can train your voice, you need to train your ear. Become sensitive to sounds and voices.

Every sound has four characteristics:

- Pitch = the highness or lowness of a sound

- Volume = the loudness of a sound

- Quality (or timbre) = the character of a sound; what makes one voice different from another

- Duration = the length of time a sound lasts

Cultivate your sensitivity to these four characteristics. Try these exercises:

Listen to a news programme. See how the presenter varies his or her voice to fit the different material; solemn news, sad news, news of international importance, light-hearted news, travel news, the weather, interviews.

Collect accents. Listen out for as many different ways of saying the same word as you can.

Listen to someone whose voice you like. Then listen to someone whose voice you find ugly. Try to identify what it is about each of the voices that you like or dislike.

LISTEN TO YOURSELF

When you've got used to listening to other people, start listening to yourself. Tape record yourself talking and reading out loud. Include your name and some bits of your speech – the whole thing if you like. Then listen really hard with your newly trained ear.

First, listen straight through, without stopping the tape or taking notes. What is your overall impression? Then listen again, this time in a more detailed way. Concentrate on:

- 'ums', 'ahs' and 'likes', etc.

- how you pace your speech

- how you pitch your speech

- where you place your emphasis

- how clearly you say the words

- how fluent you sound

Analyse what you hear and compare the elements with those of the person whose voice you admiringly listened to in the previous exercise. Ask a number of other people what they think of your voice and see if there is any common ground in their answers.

Listen to your voice as you speak and when you make those verbal tics you identified in the first exercise. Is it when you're tired? Or nervous? Or speaking to specific people?

WORK ON YOUR VOICE

So many of our verbal characteristics are learned – how we speak defines us in society. If you went to public school, you've probably got a posh accent and people will judge you according to their own preconceptions of posh people. And vice versa, if you grew up on a council estate in the East End of London. If by some quirk of fate you'd moved to the other end of the country when you were three years old, you would have a different speaking voice today.

You need to free your voice – to explore what your voice is capable of. So have fun with the following (in the privacy of your own home!):

VOICE EXERCISES

1 Make animal noises.

2 Imitate musical sounds – really try to make your voice sound like an instrument. Say 'ding' like a bell, letting the 'ng' die out very slowly.

3 Try saying these words in as many different ways as you can: Good morning, Hello, Yes, No.

4 Count out loud. As you say each number, make it sound different from the one before – louder, softer, more high-pitched, deeper. Try injecting emotion into the numbers – sound excited for one, solemn for the next, and so on.

HOW CAN I MAKE MY WORDS SOUND MORE INTERESTING?

We all know that monotonous speakers are dull, boring and hard to listen to – even if the listener is really *trying* to pay attention.

Most of us have interesting voices, complete with light and shade, varied pitch and modulation and changes in speed. We just don't realise we're doing it, because we're not thinking about speaking, we're just talking.

So when we stand up to speak in public, we suddenly realise everyone's listening to us; we get all self-conscious and the interesting voice disappears, to be replaced by a nervous, shaky monotone.

You've worked on your voice. Now for a few tips on making your words sound more interesting at all times.

BE CHATTY If you prepare for your big speech by watching tapes of Winston Churchill, Hitler or Mussolini addressing vast crowds of people, you might end up sounding like a pompous fool when you finally take to the stage. Unless, of course, you *are* speaking to vast crowds of people and the purpose of your speech is to inspire them to revolution or something. In which case, I'm highly flattered that you're reading this book, and can I have a seat in your new government? Or an important honour, at the very least?

Assuming you're not the next Fidel Castro, or leading your people to freedom from an evil dictator, I'd advise you to develop the chatty kind of style adopted almost universally by modern speakers.

If we're talking world leaders, the conversational style of speaking was good enough for Franklin D Roosevelt, who made it his personal trademark and used it in his famous 'fireside chats', intended to make radio audiences feel he was in their living-rooms with them. (Quite a scary thought, actually!)

So if it was good enough for Roosevelt, it's good enough for us. Practise reading your speech until you're really familiar with it. Avoid trying to speak written English (see chapter 3) and speak as you normally would – only a bit more clearly.

>> p27
Scripts versus cue cards

Apparently, the optimum speed to deliver speeches is around 150 to 200 words per minute. Which is little help really. Well, if you can be bothered to count out 200 words and time yourself until they fit into a minute, that's up to you. If you really have

a tendency to gabble, it might be a worthwhile exercise. For me, life's too short and I think I'd forget it all when the nerves took over anyway. Personally, I think it's more useful to tackle the nerves that make you gabble in the first place.

>> p41

Think about rhythm & flow

CHANGE THE PACE If you paid attention in chapter 3, you should have written a few changes of pace into your speech already. We looked at how changes in rhythm keep the attention of the audience.

You can maximise this effect by thinking about your subject-matter, and varying your pace accordingly. Speed up when you're talking about exciting things and slow down when you get to more serious points.

If you find the adrenalin is making you gabble, despite your relaxation exercises, remember to take a deep breath before a new sentence and to pause for a second before a new paragraph. It will stop the gabble and will reinvigorate your lungs, making your voice sound more powerful.

CHANGE THE PITCH Equally, we all have the capacity to make our voice louder and softer. So in those speedy, exciting bits, you can also raise your voice. You could even practise dropping your voice to a 'stage' whisper – it will make people lean forward to hear you and increase the atmosphere in the room.

If you're feeling particularly mischievous, you might carry on lowering and lowering your voice until the room is very quiet indeed. And then shock them by suddenly bellowing really loudly. It will raise a laugh and wake up anyone who was getting a bit sleepy. But don't do it if you're making the annual address at the Heart Transplant Patients' Society. It won't be funny.

SHUT UP ALTOGETHER You can also use pauses to help add rhythm and emphasis to your presentation. You're probably standing there, bombarding them with new information. If you don't give them a few moments of silence, they won't be able to assimilate what you're saying.

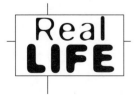

I commute to my office and use the time on the train to catch up on my reading. Often, I find myself staring out of the window. It's not because the book is boring – quite the opposite. I like to savour a particularly interesting

point and turn it over in my mind. That's the reading equivalent of silence during a speech.

If you want to emphasise a point, try pausing for a second or two.

To move onto a new point altogether, pause for longer – about four seconds, or whatever feels comfortable. It will signal the fact that one point is ending and it will help the audience make the mental leap to the new topic.

BE CRYSTAL CLEAR It doesn't matter if you have an accent; what does matter is making your words clear. If you're out of breath before you've get to the end of long words, you're gabbling and you need to slow down.

GENERAL TIPS FOR SPEAKING DURING THE PRESENTATION

DO remember the easiest and most important thing: speak up and never mumble.

DO smile, if it's appropriate. It makes your voice sound more animated. If you're talking about something serious, then don't sit there like a grinning popinjay. (You've probably already worked that out for yourself.)

DO concentrate on meaning. Open a book at a random page, read a passage and concentrate on what it's trying to say. Then read it aloud.

Here are a few trade secrets that can help everyone make a difference to their voice:

1 Speak clearly and avoid filling pauses with 'uh', 'um' and 'you know', etc.

2 Vary your pitch and speaking speed – it will keep the audience interested.

3 If there's no microphone and you have a fairly large room, make sure you project your voice clearly. Speak from the chest, not the throat.

4 Pause slightly before important points, so that the audience can mentally prepare for them.

5 If you stumble over a word, take that as a sign that you need to slow down.

WHAT SHOULD I DO WITH MY BODY?

HOW SHOULD I STAND?

Start off by standing in a relaxed and balanced way. Spread your weight over both feet, with your toes and heels on the ground. Keep your knees slightly relaxed. Take a deep breath – lower and loosen your shoulders. Beware of unconscious rocking or swaying.

MOVING AROUND

Feel free to move around the stage if it suits you. But avoid moving in a set pattern or it will look like you're doing the tango.

Moving from side to side is more effective at ringing the changes than moving backwards and forwards because, if the room is large, it can affect the perspective. You may have noticed this when watching television. The moving camera that the runners are effectively running towards makes it look as if the athlete in second place is right on the winner's heels. But the camera at the side of the track shows there's a much bigger gap between them.

ILLUSTRATION 11:   Moving from side to side is fine but avoid swaying

When you finish, thank the audience, gather together your papers and exit with aplomb!

GESTURES

The question of what to do with your hands is one that exercises fledgling public speakers out of all proportion to its importance.

You think back to other times when you've got up to say a few words and suddenly you've morphed into that Kenny Everett character who had enormous whirling hands.

You become aware that all eyes in the room are on you and every fear you've ever had of being clumsy and uncool comes rushing back to you, and every move you make seems meaningless, over the top and totally uncontrollable.

The problem is, delivering a speech isn't a dance routine. You can't choreograph gestures; if you try, they will look unnatural and unconvincing. But I'm not going to leave it at that and send you up to the lectern trembling because you feel like you're wearing somebody else's arms. Although you can't plan your gestures, there *are* some hints and tips to help you control your body and feel less self-conscious.

DO start with your hands together. That gets over the problem at the very beginning. As you begin to speak, you may forget your awkwardness and your hands will naturally move around and then come back together.

DO hold on to the lectern if there is one – but loosely! Don't grip so tightly that you can't loosen your grip and the audience can see your knuckles turn white. To avoid the temptation to grip, it's better to rest your hands lightly on the lectern.

DO use a desk if it's there. You can try placing your hands on top of it – but only if it's the right height. Don't feel you have to hunch over, just so that you can touch the table.

DO hold your notes if you're standing in the middle of the room with nothing in front of you – that will give you something to do with your hands. It will look slightly more professional to have your note cards on a table nearby – although this leaves you again with the problem of what to do with your hands.

DO create opportunities to gesture by using phrases such as 'on the one hand ... on the other'. You can also count on your fingers if you've numbered your points.

Different venues call for different gestures. Cinema actors pare down their gestures almost to nothing, because the camera does much of the work for them. By zooming in close, a face – or even part of a face – can fill an entire cinema screen, making a raised eyebrow speak louder than any words. When such actors transfer to the stage (as seems to be the trend for Hollywood stars at the moment), they often have problems making their gestures 'big' enough for the audience to notice. All that 'internal' acting is no good if the person sitting at the back of the Upper Circle doesn't realise that the actor is having a seminal moment.

The same principle can be applied to public speaking. If you're in a small meeting-room at the office, keep your gestures fairly small. Motion with your hands and forearms, bending your arms at the elbows. But if you're in a huge conference hall, you can afford to be more theatrical. Gesture with your whole arm – go on, don't be afraid!

Gestures made above elbow level carry more authority than those made below elbows. To an audience, the latter will look like the physical equivalent of muttering. Making a fist and pointing a finger looks aggressive on television but in a presentation it can add passion and emphasis.

Ask your friends what gestures you make when you're nervous. If they say you always fiddle with your hair or jingle your pocket change, make sure you avoid these movements during the presentation. If possible, take the temptation away – tie your hair back and empty your pockets.

Once you think you've got it sorted, videotape yourself and watch it back with the sound turned off. Watch carefully – most of your nervousness won't even show! But if there are any awkward gestures, make a mental note to avoid doing them. Keep the thought throughout the next few days, while in the office and at home. If you find yourself making the action, stop yourself. When you've stopped worrying that you look ugly or fat, once you've watched yourself on tape, you'll probably feel better.

ESTABLISHING CONTACT WITH THE AUDIENCE

If you're only speaking to a few people, don't sit at the table shuffling your notes and pretending you can't see them as they arrive. Get up and shake hands as they enter, sit them down, make sure they're comfortable. You'll be at an advantage before you even start.

If you're speaking to a larger audience, approach the stage (if there is one) with confidence. Smile as you introduce yourself or your speech.

Establish eye contact with the audience, including those lurking at the back.

If maintaining direct eye contact makes you feel uncomfortable, look at noses. They won't notice the difference. Get someone to try it on you, if you're sceptical.

During the presentation itself, when you've finished with a card, don't put it down on the table, put it to the back of the stack in your hand. That way the audience won't be distracted by trying to work out how long there is to go, whether you've got more cards in your hand or on the table!

That's it – everything's now in place. Breathe, relax. And deliver the killer presentation!

SUMMARY

I hope you're now feeling a little better about the personal element of the presentation. Let's recap:

Nerves – schmerves!

Kill the fear but deal with any nerves that persist.

Make yourself clear

Become a listener and remember that your aim is simply to be understood.

Control those bodyparts

Practise what you're going to do with all those arms and legs.

You and the audience

Meet, greet and act human.

7
TIME FOR
QUESTIONS

* THE PROS & CONS OF TAKING QUESTIONS

* PREPARING FOR QUESTIONS

* STAYING IN CONTROL

* DEALING WITH DIFFICULT PEOPLE

You've sorted out the speech, worked out the visuals, ironed out your verbal and physical tics, checked out the venue and you know the workings of your equipment so well that you're considering setting up as an engineer. Home and dry then, yes?

Well, no. There's still Question Time to contend with. If you don't have the ferocity, confidence and mental agility of Jeremy Paxman, you're probably a bit nervous about taking questions. It's understandable.

So skip it altogether then, yes? Scrap the Question Time. Ramble on until it's time for the coffee break and avoid the issue. Well, it's an option, but let's examine the situation first.

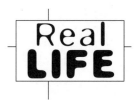

James Scott is a successful marketing manager – so successful, in fact, that he's often asked to speak at conferences and seminars.

James enjoys researching and delivering his presentations, but he dreads the moment when he has to throw the subject open for questions.

He says: 'I prepare like a loony for the presentation itself but once I allow someone else to speak, anything can happen. This is when I might really dry up. Someone might use it as an opportunity to take a pop at me. They might ask something really difficult that I just can't answer. They might go on and on and I won't be able to stop them.'

THE PROS & CONS OF TAKING QUESTIONS

Is it a short speech just to welcome, or close a meeting? Is it an informal speech – reminding your family why they're here to celebrate Granny's 90th birthday? If so, questions obviously aren't appropriate.

You might also think about scrapping the idea if you're speaking to a really huge audience. There's nothing worse than opening up for questions only to be met with a stony silence because everyone's too afraid to speak up. (Although there is a way round this – but we'll get on to it later.)

But if your presentation is controversial, complicated or (as it should be) a matter close to the audience's heart, they're bound to want to ask questions. If you're speaking at a conference, people may have paid hundreds of pounds to be there – and they want to get their money's worth. If they wanted to be talked *at*, they could have bought a video.

Question Time should be an opportunity to get in touch with the audience's opinions or feelings. If they have questions, or reservations, Question Time should root them out and give you the chance to convince them to buy your product/join your campaign/agree with your argument.

We discussed earlier that audiences have a limited attention span. If you've been banging on for a while, announcing Question Time will perk them up no end – even if it's because they're going to hear someone else's voice, or because they know they'll be able to go to the loo in ten minutes.

There are all kinds of good reasons for taking questions – let's summarise them:

1 You can communicate directly with your audience.

2 It offers a change of pace, boosting attention.

3 Handle it well and they'll admire you more.

4 You can clarify anything that you didn't communicate clearly enough.

5 You can find out exactly what's on their minds.

PREPARING FOR QUESTIONS

You can't prepare for questions, can you? You have no idea what people might ask! Wrong. You can't predict every possible one, but if you do a bit of work you can guess at several likely questions.

Depending on the subject-matter, people are most likely to ask:

● What's the first thing we should do?

● What will we get out of it?

● What if we don't do this?

● What should we do about this?

● How long will this take?

● What about the financial side of it?

Apply these questions to your own topic and think about how you might answer them.

If you're not confident about speaking off the cuff, jot down some notes. The audience won't mind – they'll just think you're really well prepared.

BRAINSTORM QUESTIONS!

Persuade, bully or bribe someone suitable to listen to you rehearse your speech. Don't ask them when they're in a rush – block out some time in their diary, even if it's your partner. Tell them you really need their help and appreciate their input. Then run through the presentation and spend an hour or so brainstorming questions. Don't let them interrupt – give them a pen and paper, so they can jot things down as they occur to them. If you can persuade family members to pay attention, they're often the best test audiences – because they can be brutally critical!

If there's any chance of getting two or three people to listen and brainstorm, so much the better. They'll bounce ideas off each other and the session will be more effective.

PLANTING QUESTIONS

Of course, one way of making sure you're fully prepared for questions is to plant some! You might be shocked at this; it seems a bit like cheating, doesn't it?

But most speakers routinely plant questions, asking someone they trust from the audience to open Question Time with a particular query. It can mean avoiding an embarrassing silence.

Not only will it make you look good when you answer the question confidently, but you'll make the audience feel better too. They might be burning with questions, but many will be too shy to be the first to put their hand up. Planting questions helps to break the ice.

GETTING BACK-UP

You might be really nervous about answering detailed questions. If so, it's fine to invite someone else along to provide backup. Don't hide the fact! Finish the main body of your speech and say:

'Right, now let me have a quick slurp of water and give you the chance to have your say. Feel free to ask any questions you like. I've asked John from marketing and Brenda from sales to come along and help out if we stray into their areas of expertise.'

Then if such a question does pop up, simply say:

'Well, I've got my own views about that, but John can really tell us what marketing makes of it. John?'

If you do draft in some 'experts' and there's not a separate chairperson for the meeting, remember that you're still in charge and will be expected to control the session (of which, more next).

Throughout Question Time, remember your Objective. Don't stray too far from your Mind Map.

STAYING IN CONTROL

When you kick off your speech, tell the audience that you will be allowing five minutes for questions at the end of the presentation.

If you anticipate lots of questions, allow more time – the audience will feel frustrated if you talk for hours but their questions have to be cut short.

SIGNAL A CHANGE As we found above, the audience will perk up when you announce it's time for questions. Make the most of this by changing the feel of the presentation. You might want to sit down, or wander about more. At the least, pour a glass of water and take a deep breath. Use that change of pace to relax and reinvigorate the presentation.

DO make sure you listen to what your questioner is asking. Sometimes it's a good idea to repeat the question.

DO make sure you've understood it.

DO make sure the rest of the audience has heard it.

DO diffuse aggressive questions. If you're asked, 'Why should I waste time and money asking the council for traffic calming, when we all know it won't do any good,' paraphrase this by saying, 'So, you want to know if the council will really pay any attention to our campaign.'

DO give yourself a few moments to think how you'd like to respond.

But DON'T repeat the question at smaller or more informal meetings. It can become an annoying habit!

PAUSE BEFORE ANSWERING Give yourself a few moments to think. The audience won't mind: it will seem like a much longer pause to you than to them, and they'll think you're taking the question very seriously. From your point of view, it will give you time to think of an answer that's relevant, concise and considered.

INVOLVE THEM You might want to welcome questions, saying 'That's a good point' or 'What an interesting angle'. When answering, start off by making eye contact with the questioner and addressing your remarks to them, but then move out and try to involve every-body. 'We can see why Jane has raised that particular point …'

IS THE QUESTIONER HAPPY? Finish each answer by going back to the questioner and asking 'Does that answer your question?' or similar. Make sure they're happy. If they're not, the following section might help you more.

KEEP AN EYE ON THE TIME If you've said you're going to allow ten minutes for questions, allow ten minutes. If you're meant to finish at 12.30, stop your speech at 12.20 and open the question session. Then keep a close eye on the time. You may want to take off your watch and put it on the desk in front of you.

DO make sure the audience knows you're still in charge.

DO say, a couple of minutes before the end, something like: **'We've just got time for one final question before we break for lunch.' The audience will know they need to keep it brief – especially if they can hear stomachs rumbling!**

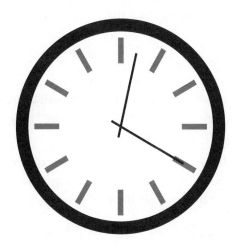

ILLUSTRATION 12:   Make sure you have a watch or clock in easy sight

BE FLEXIBLE! If the questions are coming thick and fast, the audience is obviously keen to continue for a while. You could say: 'Well, I have time for a couple more questions, if you'd like to extend this for a minute or two.'

FINISH ON A HIGH NOTE If you've just delivered a brilliant answer but there's still a minute on the clock, quit while you're ahead and jump straight to your closing comments. If, on the other hand, you've limped through a pathetic explanation, simply keep them there for another minute or so, while you take another question. Try to finish strongly!

DEALING WITH DIFFICULT PEOPLE

Ah, the thing that speakers fear the most: the Difficult Questioner.

Sometimes people don't mean to be difficult – they just stray off the point, or stumble into a sensitive issue. They might even be right on the money, but they've come up with an issue you hadn't even considered and have no idea how to answer. If this is the case, you have a number of options:

If you brought along back-up, now's the time to toss the question over. Or if you know there's someone else in the room who's likely to have the answer, draw them in. It's fine to say: 'Thanks George, I hadn't considered that before. I can see our head of human resources, Angela Owens, at the back of the room. Perhaps Angela can shed some light on the question?' Or you might even throw the question open to the floor: 'I'm sorry, I don't know the answer to that. Is there anyone here who does?'

You can also admit you don't know but whatever you do, don't waffle. The audience will see through it straight away and you'll lose any respect you built up during your speech.

DO say: 'Well, George, you've got me there. I've never looked into that aspect of it before. But it's a valuable point and I'll do my best to find out and get back to you this afternoon.'

DO get back to him, if you say you will.

DO shoot the question back: 'I don't know, I've never thought about that. Why do you ask?'

DO consider whether the question is relevant to your

presentation. If not, suggest you discuss it after the speech.

DON'T worry if you don't know everything – be confident. No one can be expected to know everything.

But you do get the odd audience member who simply wants to cause trouble. These usually fall into the following beasts:

1 The Show-off

2 The Wanderer

3 The Time-waster

4 The Antagonist

5 The Doubter

There's no need to panic. It's easy to stay in control, even in the face of the most Difficult Questioner. You just need to find out the nature of the beast and have a plan.

Who are the people most used to public speaking, those we see regularly on our TV screens? Do you want to phone a friend? Yes, it's politicians!

And what are politicians famous for? No chance to go 50/50 here. Yes, you've won a million – *they don't answer the questions*.

Remember – if you don't want to answer a question, you don't have to. Tell the Difficult Questioner it's not within the boundaries of what you're trying to do in this session. Tell them you don't have time to answer that right now. Tell them you'll discuss it with them later – I bet you find they're not so keen to discuss it when there's no one to hear their points and when everyone has already gone to the bar.

Let's look at the beasts we identified above.

1 **THE SHOW OFF** Distinguishing characteristics: Tends to waffle on for hours without actually having a question to ask. Can be a fighter who tries to score points by making himself look cleverer than you.

How to snare him: Stop him in his tracks. You're the one who's been asked to speak, not him. Tell him: 'Yes, Ivan, you're right. The system does have its foibles.' Don't let him drag you into a battle where you both try to prove who knows the most. Tell him he's very clever, then move on to something more interesting.

2 THE WANDERER Distinguishing characteristics: Seems intent on wandering off your Map and into the wilderness. May be well-meaning but she's taking the focus out of your presentation.

How to snare her: Steer her back on course. Tell her: 'As I said before, we only have scope to cover A, B and C in this session. If you want to talk about D, I'd be happy to discuss it with you after the session – or maybe we can set up a follow-up meeting to cover these issues.'

3 THE TIME-WASTER Distinguishing characteristics: Similar in appearance to the Wanderer, but more dangerous, because he's definitely doing it on purpose.

How to snare him: As for the Wanderer, but you might need to be firmer. If he's taking the focus away from your Objective, stop him! Say: 'Sorry, but we're a little short of time – can we have your question please?'

Say you're going to move on and take another question. If he still won't shut up, tell him: 'I'm clearly not going to sort this out in this session. I'd be happy to set aside some time later to discuss this. But now I must move on.'

4 THE ANTAGONIST Distinguishing characteristics: A particularly dangerous beast, she seems determined to disagree with you.

How to snare her: Try to play down your differences and concentrate on what you have in common. Suggest she may have misunderstood. If she gets personal, you might have to warn her to concentrate on the issues, not on any personalities. If all else fails, agree to disagree and/or discuss it later and move swiftly on.

5 THE DOUBTER Distinguishing characteristics: The Doubter tries to cast doubt on your expertise or your argument.

How to snare him: Don't pretend. Be confident enough to admit your limits. If you can, say you'll find out and tell him later. And do it. Remember, you're in charge, you've done your research and it doesn't matter if you don't know everything.

INSULTS & PUT-DOWNS

If things get really bad and the person just won't shut up, you might venture an insult or a put-down, although I'm not sure I'd recommend it!

Take a scan through some of these famous insults anyway – if nothing else, you can turn away and mutter them so no one can hear. It might just make you feel better!

When a true genius appears in this world, you may know him by this sign, that the dunces are all in confederacy against him.
Jonathan Swift

Once at a social gathering, Gladstone said to Disraeli, *I predict, Sir, that you will die either by hanging or of some vile disease.* Disraeli replied, *That all depends, Sir, upon whether I embrace your principles or your mistress.*

Has it ever occurred to you that there might be a difference between having an open mind and having holes in one's head? Richard Schultz

A cynic is a person who knows the price of everything and the value of nothing. Oscar Wilde

Don't be humble, you're not that great. Golda Meir

Every great thinker is someone else's moron. Umberto Eco

Let us be thankful for the fools. But for them the rest of us could not succeed. Mark Twain

Hating something is too much work to do. What you want to do is ignore something. It is more effective. Sridhar Ramaswamy

Never mistake motion for action. Ernest Hemingway

Only two things are infinite; the universe and human stupidity, and I'm not sure about the former. Albert Einstein

I do not want people to be agreeable, as it saves me the trouble of liking them. Jane Austen

During his 1956 presidential campaign, a woman called out to Adlai E Stevenson: *'Senator, you have the vote of every thinking person.'*

Stevenson called back: *'That's not enough madam, we need a majority.'*

Wisdom eventually comes to all of us. Someday it might even be your turn.

David and Leigh Eddings

If men's minds were like dominoes, surely his would be the double blank.

P G Wodehouse

I've had a perfectly wonderful evening. But this wasn't it.

Groucho Marx

Gentlemen, Chicolini here may talk like an idiot and look like an idiot, but don't let that fool you; he really is an idiot.   Groucho Marx

Don't say yes until I finish talking.   Darryl F Zanuck

The trouble with her is that she lacks the power of conversation, but not the power of speech.   George Bernard Shaw

I would like to take you seriously, but to do so would be an affront to your intelligence.   George Bernard Shaw

If this is tea, please bring me some coffee … but if this is coffee, please bring me some tea   Abraham Lincoln

Never interrupt your enemy when he is making a mistake.

Napoleon Bonaparte

It's always easier to quote something that someone else has said, than to have the courage to say something original.   Virginia Frans

BUT above all, try not to worry. All that sounds very scary, but most people are perfectly straightforward and they will raise their hands, ask interesting questions and let you answer and move on.

CLOSING THE QUESTION SESSION

When preparing your presentation, you'll have worked out your killer ending: the climax to the speech. But if you're going to have questions, you'll need to work out a few more closing remarks, to say *after* Question Time.

These can give you another good opportunity to reinforce your main points. If you're stuck, you can use a cut-down version of your Big Finish. Try to give yourself enough flexibility to include points raised during question time, if you can.

You might want to look at your watch and say:

'Well, we're pretty much out of time now. Thank you so much for listening – and for your thought-provoking questions. Don't forget – if we all work together and take these few simple steps, it could make all the difference to the future of our village.'

Make your ending strong, relevant and appropriate. Don't let your speech limp to a close.

SUMMARY

You've discovered that there's actually a lot you can do to get ready for the question session. Let's recap:

Prepare for questions

Get ready for the most frequently asked questions and guess the rest.

You're in control

Learn the expert tips on dealing with Question Time – the final furlong.

Different people and hecklers

Master the art of keeping the upper hand.

8

SPECIAL

SPECIAL
SPEECHES

* **BUSINESS PRESENTATIONS**

* **HIGHLY FORMAL SPEECHES**

* **SPEAKING OFF THE CUFF**

Some forms of public speaking have a special structure and, while these can vary quite a bit, this section should help to prepare you for tackling what can be rather imposing situations.

Like all speeches or presentations, you must always have a clear idea of what your Objective is from the outset. The structure of the meeting or presentation will then dictate how you tailor your speech to suit.

The key is to stay in control, if not of the entire event, then at least of your contribution to the proceedings. Be clear about what you want to say and put your message across in a logical manner and you won't go far wrong.

BUSINESS PRESENTATIONS

The tips for public speaking in general can usually be applied to business presentations – indeed business presentations are often easier to deliver, because your Objective is usually clear from the start and you already have some familiarity with the subject-matter.

Broadly, business presentations have one of three main aims:

1 **TO PERSUADE** The majority of business presentations are aimed at persuading the audience. Sales presentations and pitches fall into this category, but it also includes product launches and talks when you need to challenge a point of view.

2 **TO INFORM** This kind of presentation is fairly straightforward. It's the presentation of factual material. You might be inducting new recruits to your company, or presenting company results.

3 **TO INSTRUCT** This takes the second step an stage further. It is intended to give the audience new information or skills plus the ability to use it. Training sessions fall into this category.

When establishing your Objective – to sell your product, inform staff about health and safety procedures or to teach the new accounting system to the department – you should also bear in mind which category your presentation falls into.

THE BRIEF

If you've been asked to give the presentation, you will have been given some kind of brief. This might have come from your boss, a different department, or from the client herself.

You might not even realise you've had a brief – it's not necessarily a detailed document; it could be an email, a phone call or a chat in the corridor.

Rewrite the brief in your own words and send it to the person who's asked you to present. This will ensure, at an early stage, that you understand exactly what's required, and it will show your commitment to giving the presentation you really want. It can be done in the form of a letter, an email, an agenda, a memo – whatever you feel is most appropriate.

This is the time to include any questions about the brief.

Your confirmation might look like this:

MEMO

From: Greg Dempsey, development

To: Janet Smith, press office

Re: Demonstration of new meal range

Janet,

Just a note to confirm that I have booked the first-floor meeting-room for 12.30 on Wednesday 6 September for the meeting to show you the new meal range, so that you are well-prepared for the planned launch on 15 January.

I know you haven't been told much about this yet, so I anticipate the presentation will take about an hour – we intend to talk you through the story behind the new recipes (we have a five-minute slide-show to help with this), before we start sampling the dishes. Of course, we should be able to answer any other questions as we go along.

I will head the demonstration, with Dean Ambrose and Gemma Bonham explaining the development of the projects.

I understand that you, Joy and Simone will be attending from your department – do you think we should invite Carol Jones from Marketing?

Give me a call on extension 6831 if you have any further questions.

Greg

ILLUSTRATION 13:   Maintaining communication is essential to make sure everything runs smoothly

You should also write a memo for yourself, so you don't forget that you promised to email everyone to tell them where the meeting is being held. This memo should then be copied to everyone involved – including your boss – to keep them informed.

CHECKLIST

Checklist for confirming a brief

Ask yourself, have I confirmed:

the Objective? ❏

the End Result? ❏

what the audience expects to see and hear? ❏

the level of audience knowledge about the subject? ❏

the estimated size of audience? ❏

the timing and structure of the presentation? ❏

the venue? ❏

the date? ❏

the time (arrival time and start time, if different)? ❏

the name of the presenter/names of the presentation team? ❏

breakdown of everyone's responsibilities
    (including those of the client)? ❏

a note of the visual aids you intend, or would like, to use? ❏

PREDICT ANY PROBLEMS

Even if you're utterly clear about your brief, there might still be a few tricky issues lurking around – that's business!

Ask yourself the following questions:

● Is this presentation a test for me? Does my promotion/ assessment depend on it?

● Is this presentation particularly important for my boss? Will her job be affected by how well I do?

● What will the business get out of this? In the long term? In the short term?

● Is there anyone in the audience who might be difficult? Why? Can I do anything about it?

● Does the presentation include bad or controversial news? Why am I presenting it? How can I present it without associating the bad news with my own performance?

TALKING MONEY

Business presentations are more likely than other speeches to have a budget attached to them. Set this budget at an early stage; if there isn't a budget, costs can easily spiral out of control.

Consider the following costs when making a budget:

Room hire	❑
Hire of equipment	❑
Training	❑
Preparation of visuals (including photography, commissioning illustrations and printing handouts)	❑
Research costs (external researchers, photographic agencies, etc., will charge for research)	❑
Travel	❑
Accommodation	❑
Entertaining/catering	❑

At the same time, think about the value of the whole presentation to your business. If you're not going to make much money out of it, keep the budget low. And there's no point in your colleagues spending hours preparing for a minor presentation – their time has a cost attached to it too.

pitch before you've even started) and catering. If you're after someone's money, make sure they're fed and watered. Keep it simple but buy the best.

TROUBLESHOOTING

For important presentations, plan ahead for any possible emergencies. Think about potential problems early on in the project. In fact, write some time into your schedule to give this proper consideration. Here are some possible problems and suggested solutions.

1 **A VITAL MEMBER OF MY PRESENTATION TEAM HAS FALLEN ILL** This demonstrates the importance of working as a team, and keeping the team fully informed. Make sure notes are kept in neat, clear files, so that another member of the team can step in, if necessary. When you allocate jobs to the members of the team, also assign them as understudies to other jobs. Let the client know if someone is a stand-in, as a matter of courtesy.

2 **MY EQUIPMENT HAS BROKEN DOWN** Handouts can come into their own in this situation. Instead of giving them out at the end, hand them out during the presentation and work from them.

If you're presenting to a small audience, take back-ups of your visual material in a portfolio. If there are any problems, you can present from that.

If words are important to your presentation, arrange to have a flip chart or whiteboard there, so that you can hand-write your points.

3 **THE VENUE HAS BEEN CHANGED AT THE LAST MINUTE** Rather than panicking, find out how the change of venue impacts on your plans.

The main problem is likely to be with audiovisual equipment – either it's not provided at the new venue, or the new venue isn't suitable for what you had planned.

If it's too late to borrow or hire new equipment, fall back on the methods described above in 'My equipment has broken down'. If you've got a low-tech fall-back plan, you shouldn't go too wrong. If you had planned catering and there are no facilities at the new venue, contact a local café and ask them to deliver teas, coffees and suitable snacks. Most will be happy to do so. If you can't find anyone to do this, Marks & Spencer and Prêt à Manger both offer a sandwich delivery service.

If the change was very last-minute, the client or audience will be sympathetic to the lack of bells and whistles in your presentation.

4 **I'M STUCK IN A TRAFFIC JAM/THE TRAINS HAVE BEEN CANCELLED** Equip yourself with a mobile and all the relevant numbers before you leave. Try to allow for the vagaries of transport; if you're really early, you can always go and have a nice cup of tea first.

If you do hit problems, ring ahead, explain that there's been a crash or whatever, and give your client a realistic estimate of your arrival time. Let them know if you can shorten your presentation, and say you're extremely keen to go ahead.

5 **I HAVEN'T GOT THE RIGHT TYPE OF FURNITURE** You may have asked for tables and chairs, but that still leaves plenty of room for misunderstanding. If it's vital that you have a certain type of table (for your audiovisual equipment, for example), pop a fold-down table in the car, just in case.

6 **THERE ARE MORE PEOPLE HERE THAN I EXPECTED** Plan for this by taking extra copies of any handouts. If there are so many people that they can't see your visual aids, you can always give them a handout to use instead.

If you don't have enough handouts to go round at the end of the meeting, ask people to write their names and addresses on a sheet of paper and post on any follow-up material.

HIGHLY FORMAL SPEECHES

If you are asked to speak at a debating society, or other formal meeting, you'll need to know a bit about the complicated and old-fashioned rules that still govern this kind of thing. First of all, here is the jargon:

RULES OF ORDER

Applicable to Parliament and some formal business meetings, these are just the rules by which the meeting is governed.

THE CHAIR

Another term for the chairman of the meeting (who may or may not be a woman).

What does the chairman do? And what shouldn't he do?

- He keeps order and applies the rules of the meeting impartially.

- He avoids speaking for or against any issue. If he feels he must speak, he should vacate the chair.

- He shouldn't vote unless there's a secret ballot or he has to make the casting vote if there's a tie.

- In very formal meetings, he shouldn't say 'I', 'you' or 'we', etc., but should say things like 'Would the speakers please remember to address all comments through the Chair'. Equally, speakers should call him 'Mr Chairman' or 'the Chair'.

RISING TO BE RECOGNISED

In formal meetings, no one can get up to speak unless they are 'recognised' by the Chair. In a large meeting, this usually means you should stand up. In a smaller meeting, it's OK just to raise your hand.

Etiquette says you shouldn't interrupt another speaker to do this.

The Chairman should normally recognise speakers in the order they stood up, i.e. first come, first served.

HAVING THE FLOOR

Once you've been recognised, you 'have the floor'. That means you can speak and, under normal circumstances, no one else should interrupt.

There might be a time limit on how long you should speak. Apart from that, you can carry on as long as you are 'in order' (i.e., proper and relevant). The term 'proper' can be a bit difficult to define. But generally, remember you're in a formal situation, so you should be careful not to offend anyone.

The exception is if you're discussing an impeachment or something similar, when character judgements are necessary. But make sure anything you say would also stand up in court.

MAKING AND SECONDING MOTIONS

If the meeting has finished with everything on the agenda, and there's time for any other business, you can introduce a new topic in the form of a motion.

This is how you should do it:

YOU (MRS A): (rising to be recognised) *Mr Chairman.*

CHAIRMAN: *The Chair recognises Mrs A.*

MRS A: (Briefly explain what you want to do) *So I move that such and such be done.*

CHAIRMAN: (If he agrees this is in order) *It has been moved that such and such be done. Is there a seconder?*

MRS B: *I second the motion.*

CHAIRMAN: *It has been moved and seconded that such and such be done. Is there any discussion?*

Seconding isn't always necessary, but the reason for it is to check there's more than one person interested in a topic, before it's taken on for discussion.

ORDER OF BUSINESS/AGENDA

These are more or less the same thing but an agenda is more detailed. It sets out what the meeting is going to cover. When the meeting is underway, you must cover the topic that is currently being discussed. If you try to discuss another, it is literally 'out of order'.

Formal meetings usually go something like this:

CALL TO ORDER The chairman may rap his gavel (a wooden hammer, like that used by auctioneers) and say: *The meeting will please come to order.* This starts the meeting.

THE MINUTES The secretary records the proceedings of the meeting in a permanent record called the minutes.

Meetings usually start with the reading of the minutes of the last meeting. The secretary reads them out and the Chairman asks if the members agree with the changes.

When everyone is happy, the minutes are said to have been approved.

REPORTS Meetings may include reports by officers and committees. They are usually heard in the following order:

Officers: President, vice-president, secretary, treasurer.

Committees: Standing committees, special committees.

GENERAL ORDERS After all the reports have been read, the meeting moves on to general orders of business – motions that have been put down for discussion. For example:

Chairman: *As the first general order of business tonight we have to consider the recommendation of the Environment Committee at the last meeting that we run all Society vehicles on unleaded petrol. Is there any discussion?*

UNFINISHED BUSINESS Sometimes meetings have to close without coming to any real conclusion about a motion. This then becomes unfinished business and is taken up at the next meeting, after general orders.

NEW BUSINESS This is your chance to bring up something new. It's a good idea to jot down what you want to propose as a motion, so you don't stumble over your words. You should also discuss it beforehand with someone else, to make sure it will be seconded. A more experienced member will also be able to give you advice on how to word your proposal. If possible, speak to the Chairman before the meeting and let him know what you're planning.

Some organisations say that anyone wanting to propose a motion under new business should supply it in writing to the secretary some time before the meeting.

But if it is all right to make the proposal in the meeting, wait for the Chairman to call for new business, rise to be recognised and propose your motion, as described above.

ADJOURNMENT The meeting goes on until it is in recess or adjournment. Recess is a short break. Adjournment is the formal end of the meeting. People might still sit around and chat, but the formal bit is all over.

For more information on debating and formal speaking procedures, try **www.actein.edu.au/ACTDU/owndebate**.

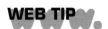

SPEAKING OFF THE CUFF

You may have been called upon to 'say a few words' at a colleague's leaving party, a family birthday party or the like. The shock of being called upon, totally unprepared, may have fazed you, and you might feel you stumbled through, sounding like an empty-headed fool.

It's trying to speak 'off the cuff' that has caused much of the general terror at the thought of speaking in public.

Even if this hasn't happened to you, we have all sat through such occasions, trying not to meet anyone's eye in case it *does* happen and one is forced to one's feet.

When you speak off the cuff, you literally make up your speech as you go along. So no chance of mind-mapping, setting an Objective or End Result, luxuriating in the pros and cons of script versus cue cards, and all the other preparation devices we've already covered.

This is true. But many of the other tips and hints included in the book will improve your performance, whether you're speaking from a prepared speech or off the cuff. If you know that your voice, stance and gestures have been considered, all you need to worry about is what you're going to say.

Speaking extemporaneously, as the dictionary would have it, *is* difficult for most people who are unaccustomed to public speaking. But some people can do it, so what's the trick?

The trick is that most of the time, they're not speaking off the cuff. Television and radio presenters may be hugely experienced wordmasters, but even when they appear to be speaking spontaneously, they might still be reading from an autocue, or performing a well-rehearsed piece. So don't punish yourself thinking that everyone else can do it.

Even if they haven't learned their speech, or don't have carefully hidden 'idiot boards' around the room, they might be using a few tricks of the trade.

The thing to remember is that there's 'off the cuff' and there's 'off the cuff'. Most of the time, you will actually have a chance to plan what you're going to say.

If a member of your staff is leaving, or you are likely to win a prize, you'll know about it in advance and you'll have a good idea that you might be asked to say a few words. Instead of burying your head in the sand and hoping it doesn't happen, take some time out to think what you *would* say, if you were asked.

Even if you have the shortest of short notices, decide your Objective in double-quick time. You might want to speak about the importance of family; the changes in the business over the years; or simply that your secretary was the best you've ever had. Keep that at the forefront of your mind, just as you would for any public speech.

If you have more time, think about your Mind Map – identify a few key points that you want to cover. Everyone knows you're speaking off the cuff, so they won't be expecting miracles.

Consider the following structure:

● State your Objective – your key message.

● Expand on it.

● Tell a story or give examples to illustrate your Objective.

● Return to your Objective, saying it in a different way – possibly with added strength.

● Shut up.

DON'T waffle on.

DO what you're asked: say a few words.

One high-profile example of an unrehearsed speech is Robert F Kennedy's eulogy to Martin Luther King Jr. King was assassinated in Memphis on 5 April 1968, just as Kennedy – then a candidate in the Indiana presidential primary – was on a plane to Indianapolis. He was due to speak on the tarmac to a group of people, who were already there, awaiting his arrival. The audience had no idea that King had been killed, but Kennedy heard the news mid-flight. He junked his prepared words and, on arrival, delivered the speech of his life.

Another famed – but underrated – off the cuff speaker is the former Labour Party leader, Neil Kinnock. His Welsh articulateness and passion failed to shine through when he was forced to deliver the carefully worded speeches written by advisors who, having been in Opposition for some time, were more afraid of upsetting voters than

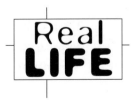

anything else. But when Kinnock was given a free reign, he produced his best speeches. One such was delivered to the Welsh Labour Party at Llandudno on 15 May 1987. The following passage became the best known of the speech – see what dynamic language he chooses and how his words are based on normal, natural speech patterns:

Why am I the first Kinnock in a thousand generations to be able to get to university? Why is Glenys the first woman in her family in a thousand generations to be able to get to university?

Was it because all our predecessors were 'thick'? Did they lack talent – those people who could sing, and play, and recite and write poetry; those people who could make wonderful, beautiful things with their hands; those people who could dream dreams, see visions; those people who had such a sense of perception as to know in times so brutal, so oppressive, that they could win their way out of that by coming together?

Were those people not university material? Couldn't they have knocked off all their A-levels in an afternoon?

But why didn't they get it?

Was it because they were weak? – those people who could work eight hours underground and then come up and play football?

Weak? Those women who could survive eleven childbearings, were they weak? Those people who could stand with their backs and their legs straight and face the people who had control over their lives, the ones who owned their workplaces and tried to own them, and tell them, 'No, I won't take your orders.' Were they weak?

Does anybody really think that they didn't get what we had because they didn't have the talent, or the strength, or the endurance, or the commitment?

Of course not.

Taken from The Penguin Book of Twentieth-Century Speeches.

>> p136

Speaking at weddings

WEDDINGS

Many people are called upon to speak at a wedding at one time or another – even if it's just their own. Because of this, and because of the maze of special rules that govern weddings, I've devoted an entire chapter, the following one, to the subject.

SPEAKING TO THE MEDIA

There are dozens of reasons why you might be called upon to talk to the media. Again, there are special rules and special skills involved. I have given a whole chapter to the subject, chapter 10.

>> p164

Speaking to the media

SUMMARY

Special speeches require special skills, so make sure you've run through all the sections. Let's recap:

Business presentations

Confirm the brief

Predict any problems

Set your budget

Know your audience

Work to your deadline

Create the content

Choose the venue

Troubleshooting

Formal public speaking

Familiarise yourself with all the terms and you'll be fine

Speaking off the cuff

State your Objective

Expand

Tell a story

Return to your Objective

Shut up

9

WEDDINGS

* WHO SAYS WHAT? AND WHEN?

* BREAKING FROM TRADITION

* TRICKY MATTERS

* RESEARCHING YOUR SPEECH

* SUGGESTED INTRODUCTIONS

* TOASTS

* READINGS

Although weddings are becoming more informal, family traditions vary and some people are keen to follow the conventional or 'proper' way of doing things. In order to subvert something, you first have to understand it, so we'll run through the traditional way of doing things, and then look at some alternatives.

When you think of wedding speeches, you probably think of the slightly risqué best man's speech that upsets some maiden aunt. Or of the father of the bride's speech which embarrasses the bride!

In fact, one of the main purposes of wedding speeches is to thank the various members of the wedding party. And one advantage of doing things the traditional way is that everyone who should be thanked, gets thanked.

The speeches also congratulate the newlyweds and include the toasts – and no one minds the latter!

Different cultures and faiths have different traditions – even within Britain. Irish and Scottish weddings might follow a different speech order to English weddings – and the Irish are famous for their way with words, so they tend to go on a bit longer!

It's outside the scope of this book to deal with lots of different types of wedding – a specialist publication will do that much better. So forgive me for dealing with the English wedding – the Scots, Irish and Welsh aren't usually *too* different. And if your family follows its own traditions, I'm sure the mothers of the bride and groom will be happy to volunteer any changes to the suggestions I include here!

WHO SAYS WHAT? AND WHEN?

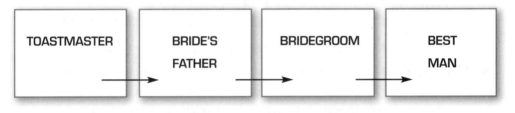

| TOASTMASTER | BRIDE'S FATHER | BRIDEGROOM | BEST MAN |

ILLUSTRATION 14   Typical order of wedding speeches

TOASTMASTER

There may be a toastmaster; if there is, he'll introduce the speeches. If not, this job falls to the best man. Whoever is doing the job simply asks for silence and introduces the first speaker.

BRIDE'S FATHER

As the first speaker, you will effectively set the scene for the rest of the speeches. Traditionally, this is because the bride's father pays for – and therefore hosts – the wedding.

Officially, you speak on behalf of your wife and yourself. A great part of your speech will be about your daughter and, although fathers and daughters are supposed to have a special relationship, try to steer clear of clichés and talk about your own relationship. Real life anecdotes say more about that relationship than any amount of generalisation about fathers and daughters. Don't be afraid to talk about the times

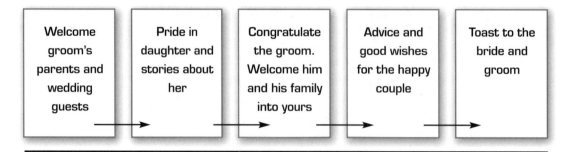

| Welcome groom's parents and wedding guests | Pride in daughter and stories about her | Congratulate the groom. Welcome him and his family into yours | Advice and good wishes for the happy couple | Toast to the bride and groom |

ILLUSTRATION 15:   Main points of the father of the bride's speech

you didn't see eye to eye – probably during her teenage years – as long as you counter this with something about how she's grown into a wonderful woman, or how you always loved each other underneath it all. Traditionally, your speech should include:

- a welcome to the groom's parents, both families and other guests – particularly if they've travelled a long way
- mention of how proud you and your wife are of your daughter
- something about the events leading up to the wedding
- some anecdotes about the bride's childhood and earlier adulthood – how she has surpassed or changed your expectations of her, how you view the strength in her relationship with her new husband
- congratulations to the groom
- something about how happy you are to get to know the groom and his family
- something expressing confidence in the couple's future together
- advice to the couple for the future
- an invitation to the other guests to wish the newly-weds well
- a toast to 'the health and happiness of the bride and groom'

You might also want to add a few words about your own relationship with the groom – how you met him, what you thought at the time, something that surprised you about him or something you have learned from him.

If the father of the bride is not there for any reason, this role is normally taken by the person who gives her away.

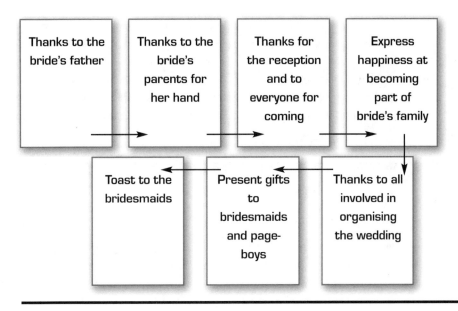

ILLUSTRATION 16:   Main points of the bridegroom's speech

BRIDEGROOM

If you're the bridegroom, you speak on behalf of your wife and yourself. This gives you the opportunity to open with the words 'My wife and I', which you can use to raise a chuckle or a bit of heckling. Don't forget that, if the bride is not speaking herself, you are speaking for the two of you. You should include:

- thanks to the bride's father for the toast

- thanks to the bride's father for his daughter's hand

- thanks for the wedding and reception

- thanks for being welcomed in to the family

- how happy you are and how lovely your bride is

- praise for the bride's parents on their daughter

- happiness at becoming part of their family

- thanks to your own parents for your upbringing

- response to the advice given by the bride's father

- any anecdotes about meeting your wife and your relationship (if the stories cast you in a slightly embarrassing light, the audience will love them even more)

- comments addressed directly to the bride about how happy you are and how much you're looking forward to the future

- thanks to guests for attending, for their good wishes and gifts

- thanks to the best man, ushers and anyone else who has helped – present them with their gifts, if you have bought gifts

- thanks to the bridesmaids and praise for their good looks

- presentation of gifts to the bridesmaids and page-boys

- a toast to 'the bridesmaids'

You might also want to include:

- further comments to the bride's father – if he has said something nice about you, you might want to return the compliment by saying how hard you'll try to fulfil his expectations, or that you are proud to be his son-in-law

- remarks about how the wedding is going – especially if anything funny has happened

- thanks to anyone else who has played a particularly important role – providing flowers, cake, food, outfits, etc.

- a few words pretending you're dreading the best man's speech but saying something nice about him (this will also act as an introduction to anyone who doesn't know him, if he hasn't already spoken)

BEST MAN

The best man has specific things to say as well as being the life and soul of the party.

If you're the best man, you're obviously meant to be hilariously funny and possessed of the public speaking skills of a major broadcaster, politician or comedian. Of that, more later. Cut down to the bone, you're supposed to respond on behalf of the bridesmaids.

You may include:

- the bridesmaids' thanks for their gifts

- your own compliments to the bridesmaids, page-boys or ushers

- admiration of the bride and something about the groom's luck in having such a lovely bride

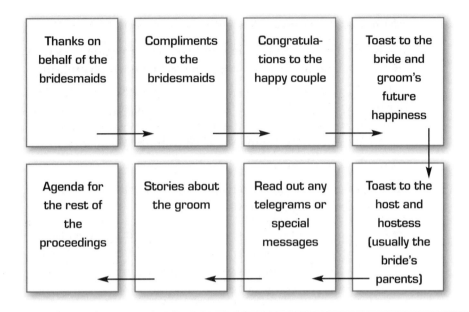

ILLUSTRATION 17:   Main points of the best man's speech

● congratulations to the happy couple

● something about being delighted to be best man

● a toast to 'The bride and groom's future happiness'

● thanks to the host and hostess on behalf of yourself and the guests

● a toast to 'The host and hostess'

● any telegrams or similar messages from guests who can't make it to the wedding

● a toast to 'Absent friends'

● stories and anecdotes about the groom – but see the special section on this!

● what's happening for the rest of the evening

A word of caution! Don't forget that this is the day on which the bride and groom have pledged their lives to each other. Also, consider the other guests. I'm not saying you have to dilute your speech so much that it wouldn't offend a Victorian spinster, but do bear in mind that there are likely to be guests of different generations, cultures and outlooks. Your risqué story might be funny down the pub, but don't risk ruining the day for anyone – especially the bride.

Mix your humour with kindness and your embarrassing tales with sincerity. Mention how you first met the groom, how you came to be such close friends, what you like and admire about him, how you viewed his relationship with the bride – mention how you first realised it was serious, or how he told you he was going to propose. You should also wish them the best for the future. You might also like to include:

● anecdotes about the wedding preparations, especially near-disasters or anything funny

● some more about the bride – try to talk to and about her as well as the groom (sometimes I think the best man would have been better off making his speech at the stag night, for all the thought he spares for the bride)

● props – I've seen a slide show (with embarrassing photos from the groom's past), a specially written song, performed by the best man and ushers, and enlarged photos, copied several times so they could be passed round the room

As I mentioned above, it can be a bit daunting to be asked to be best man at a wedding. You'll probably be speaking to a large group of people, some of whom you know and some of whom you will never have laid eyes on before. And they'll all be expecting you to be funny, warm – and audible. Quite a task.

Don't panic, you've got a number of advantages on your side:

ADVANTAGE ONE Although the best man feels the most pressure to be funny, his is usually the speech people look forward to most of all. And that goodwill can count for a lot. It's a weird phenomenon but when people know they're supposed to laugh, they usually do. How else do you explain the gales of audience laughter achieved by even the worst sitcoms on TV?

ADVANTAGE TWO If there's no toastmaster, you will have been taking control of the proceedings, giving you the advantage of already being familiar to the audience.

ADVANTAGE THREE You're on last. In the star slot. Several toasts will already have been drunk – not to mention the wine guests drank during the meal and the sips they've been taking throughout the speeches. The potential hurdles have all been overcome and everyone is now relaxing, looking forward to an evening of dancing and chatting to their friends and relatives.

So all in all, they're highly likely to greet even your lamest of gags with a roar of laughter.

BREAKING FROM TRADITION

So much for the traditional wedding. There are dozens of reasons why people choose not to stick to this format.

It might just be a matter of personal preference – the bride doesn't speak, traditionally, but many modern women are appalled by the idea of sitting quietly while the men speak on her behalf on her big day. Women who routinely chair business meetings, or pitch to high-level clients, or field questions from the media, day in, day out, might balk at the idea of the traditional, mute bride.

And the same might go for her mother. I know plenty of families where the mother is the one who sits on committees, who is a member of an amateur dramatic group, or who is simply an accomplished chatterer. Why should she sit and smile while her husband does all the talking?

THE BRIDE

The very fact that brides traditionally don't make a speech is going to free you to make the speech you want to make.

Unlike the best man and your father, you don't have years of expectation colouring what you want to say. You don't have to be uproariously funny like the best man; nor do you have to be the doting dad. But when anything goes, it's hard to know where to start.

Even though the bride's speech is a relatively recent idea, some 'new' traditions have taken root. This might be a good place to examine your thoughts about what you want to say.

The first question to tackle is *where* does your speech fit in, in the traditional order?

The father of the bride's speech is traditionally about the daughter, so if your dad is not there for any reason – or if it's been decided that he shouldn't speak – you might want to take that slot.

Or you might want to do a kind of double act with your new husband. We saw above that the groom's speech is traditionally made on behalf of himself and his new wife, so if you do want to speak, this would seem to be a logical time to do so.

However, you may prefer to let him have his say alone and keep your own words as a surprise. If this is the case, you could speak just before or just after the brand-new 'old man'.

OR (yes, there is yet another alternative), you might want to go last – although personally I think the slot after the best man is the most difficult of the evening. Give yourself a break!

Anyway, whenever you decide to do it, what do you say? Again, anything goes, really, but you might want to think about the following:

- thanks to the guests for coming, especially if they've travelled from afar

- thanks to everyone who's helped with the preparations (As traditional roles break down, more and more people get involved with the planning of a wedding and this might be a good time to thank your long-suffering best friends. After all, they've probably helped you to choose all kinds of accessories – not to mention drying your tears when you were having second thoughts about the entire thing! But best not to mention that specifically; not at the wedding!)

- a special thank-you to your mum, for helping with the wedding (if she has done so) and also for bringing you up and for your continuing relationship

- a thank-you to dad – if he's just related lots of embarrassing but heart-warming tales about you, the least you can do is to return the compliment

- a thank-you to anyone else who helped significantly with the wedding preparations

- a few words about your husband. This is your chance to put your side of the story of how you met and about any anecdotes he might be planning to tell about you. It's also the time to say something very, very nice about him

- a thank-you for any presents

- normally the groom thanks the bridesmaids but as they are your helpers on the day, it might make more sense for you to do this job

- as most wedding speeches end with a toast, the Americans have introduced a tradition that the bride proposes a toast to the guests

THE BRIDE'S MOTHER

If the bride's father is not at the wedding for some reason, his traditional role might well fall to the bride's mother. More of that below.

But what if the bride's mother *chooses* to speak – what should she say? Generally, I would advise that she sticks to a similar structure to that of the father of the bride (see above). The mother of the bride might wish to relate some tales of her own about the bride's childhood, which would give a nice, different perspective.

THE GROOM'S FATHER

The groom's family traditionally have virtually no role to play in the wedding. But many couples find this out of date – particularly if they have contributed financially to the wedding.

So you might want to consider asking the groom's father to say a very few words. He needn't say much – I would recommend that he echo the sentiments of the bride's father, thanking the latter for his welcome and saying a few words of greeting to his own family, while saying how pleased he is to meet so many members of the bride's family.

THE BEST WOMAN

Just as the best man speaks for the groom, some couples have asked the bride's best friend to perform a similar role for the bride. If you go down this route, simply review the guidelines for the best man and adapt them, as necessary.

WARNING! Having said all this, I would be wary about making speech time an opportunity for everyone to get up and have their tuppen'orth. You could go on for ever, inviting your mother's best friend's cousin to get to her feet. Don't. It's fine to dispense with tradition, but have a care for your guests. They're itching to get to the bar/chat to their favourite nephew/go to the loo/get away from their husband/chat up the bridesmaids, and they don't want to sit around the dinner-table all night.

So that's all the happy families stuff. More difficult are the situations when families don't fit in to the traditional pattern outlined above and speakers are changed not out of choice, but out of necessity. Divorce, death, adoption and stepfamilies aren't modern phenomena. But today's society is happier to acknowledge them, not to gloss over them. Which brings us on to:

TRICKY MATTERS

Of course there are still highly traditional white weddings, in which the parents are still married to each other; there are no family feuds and the bride and groom are each other's first serious partners and only just about to set up home together for the first time. Well, I suppose there are. There must be. It's just that I've never been to one. And neither has anyone I've asked.

Let's have a look at what the internet calls the FAQ (Frequently Asked Questions list):

1 What if the bride or groom has been married before?

2 Who speaks if one of the key cast is ill or dead – or has recently died?

3 What if the bride or groom has a child by a previous relationship?

4 What if parents of the bride or groom are divorced?

Weddings can be extremely difficult times. But they should be happy times. Let's have a look at those problems again and try to come up with some solutions that work in the real world – not just in the etiquette sections of the big newspapers. (See suggested intros below for speech suggestions.)

WHAT IF THE BRIDE OR GROOM HAS BEEN MARRIED BEFORE?
Whatever the circumstances, this is a difficult situation. Either partner may have been divorced or widowed, and there may or may not be children from this union.

The etiquette books will tell you that it's 'terribly bad form' to refer to any previous marriage. While I agree that one shouldn't bang on about it, eulogising about former partners or, worse, making any form of comparison whatsoever between weddings or wives, I think it's insane to ignore the facts altogether. We are no longer living in the Victorian age, when divorcees wore their status like a lifelong badge of shame. No one plans to get divorced! Yes, if that first marriage was in church, the couple swore before God that they would love and cherish, etc., 'until death us do part'. And many people still believe that breaking that promise is a sin – however it came about. But most people can see that circumstances alter cases – and they make allowances.

And anyway, the day one of those people is getting married for the second time is *not* the day for self-righteous guests to get sniffy. Apart from anything else, such a blatant triumph of hope over experience should be roundly celebrated. A divorce or bereavement is a traumatic and life-changing experience for anyone. And a first marriage was an important rite of passage, however badly things turned out or however briefly the union may have lasted. If there were children, they will presumably attend the second wedding. And children of the bride or groom are not easily ignored.

Anyway, half the guests will have brought up the issue of the first wedding anyway – usually when they're bumping into long-lost relatives and trying to remember where they last saw each other. Oh yes! It was at Jane's *last* wedding. At which point they get a bit embarrassed and tend to let those words hang in the air.

So, to get back to the point, I believe some passing reference may be made to a first marriage. It may make the guests feel more comfortable, if they know there are no secrets or taboo topics. You don't have to mention it, but if you do, be matter-of-fact and don't linger on the subject.

WHAT IF ONE OF THE KEY CAST IS ILL OR DEAD – OR HAS RECENTLY DIED?

This was the case at a wedding I recently attended. The situation was acknowledged and it was a highly emotional moment. But weddings are inherently happy occasions (on the whole), so a moment after we'd all had a lump in our throats and a tear in our eye, the speechmaker recovered with a more positive thought. And the whole speech was much the better for his honesty in mentioning a difficult subject on what is supposed to be 'the happiest day of your life'.

In the same way as divorce, illness and bereavement shouldn't be dwelt on, but should be acknowledged if the victim is an important friend or family member. If the bride's mother is a widow, the toast to the bride and groom is often made by a senior male relative (such as an uncle) or by an old family friend, who has known the bride for years. Of course, there's nothing to stop the bride's mother from stepping in and taking on the role that her late husband would have played.

If a close relative has died very recently, the family may want to pay tribute to them in some way. This can best be done before the main speeches and is most easily done by an old family friend. Close family members may want to pay tribute themselves, rather than hand the task over to a friend: if this is the case at your wedding, sit down and discuss it with them in detail. The time for long eulogies and emotion was at the funeral. Close family may take on the job with equanimity, but the highly charged atmosphere of a wedding can easily lead to too many tears.

However, you should respect their wishes and discuss the situation with consideration.

 DON'T end on a downer. Start positively, mention the sad bit, and then move on to end on a high note.

WHAT IF THE BRIDE OR GROOM HAS A CHILD BY A PREVIOUS RELATIONSHIP?

We touched on this in the question about previous marriages. Of course, there need not have been an earlier marriage for there to have been a child, but the principles remain the same. The child, in 99 per cent of cases, will be present at the wedding – and, in the majority of cases, she or he will have a special role to play: as an usher, bridesmaid or page-boy. This reflects the important status of the child and may help them to accept the wedding more happily. However, a child can be the happiest bridesmaid in the land, but if Daddy doesn't mention her in his speech, she'll swiftly transform into the unhappiest. In addition, while most of the guests will be aware of the situation, there may well be some who do not.

For both these reasons, and more, it's best to mention the child in a positive and welcoming way. We saw above how many of the speeches are meant to welcome newcomers into each other's family; the child of a couple who are no longer together should be granted the courtesy of even more welcoming into what really will be their new family.

WHAT IF THE PARENTS OF THE BRIDE OR GROOM ARE DIVORCED?

Again, this was the case at one of the weddings I attended last year. Neither the bride's nor the groom's parents were still together. And while the various relationships between them had been highly strained at times over the years, they all handled it beautifully. And the bride, who had been particularly concerned, was able to enjoy her day in exactly the right way.

If the bride's parents are divorced and a stepfather played an important role in her upbringing, a wedding can be a difficult time. Assuming that both men are to be at the wedding, many brides recoil in horror at the thought of having to choose who will 'give them away' and make a speech. One way round this would be for the bride's mother to make the speech. If she doesn't feel comfortable with this, you might want to skip the speechy bit and the mother could simply propose the toast to the bride and bridegroom.

RESEARCHING YOUR SPEECH

If you've been asked to make a speech at a wedding, the chances are that you know the bride and groom well. However, this is not always the case – you could be standing in for someone else, or for other reasons you might know one half of the couple and not the other.

Whether you think you know them well or not, it's always worth doing a bit of research. You might uncover funny or tender stories that you had never heard before.

ASK FRIENDS AND FAMILY

Make a point of calling those close to the couple and asking for their special memories. Most people will be chuffed to have been asked to help, particularly if they're not making a speech themselves. Don't expect them to have a supply of anecdotes that they can trot out like a list. You'll probably need to chat to them to draw out the best stories.

A good method is to get friends and family together over a bottle of wine. Forgotten anecdotes will be remembered and they, in turn, will prompt other stories. Take a dictaphone or tape recorder, so that you don't have to sit there frantically scribbling notes. If you're the best man (or best woman) and the groom (or bride) has a very close circle of friends, it's a nice touch to mention the other members of the gang. The same goes for aunties, uncles, cousins or grandparents.

OTHER PEOPLE

It might take a bit more work, but if you can track down old teachers or schoolfriends, former colleagues and ex-bosses, you can open the floodgates for even more stories.

FAMILY ARCHIVE

Plunder old photo albums, letters, press cuttings and school books. Childhood essays about 'what I did in the summer holidays', 'what I want to be when I grow up' or 'what I would do if I was prime minister' can often prove to be rich pickings. Take the book along to the wedding and read it out verbatim. Friends and relatives may love the chance to look at the rest of the book, later on in the evening.

Borrow photos and have copies made, to show at the wedding. Refer to old press cuttings – usually for sporting or school achievements; these can be hilarious in the light of the way the subject's life has panned out since.

ANCIENT HISTORY

Get hold of a newspaper printed the day the subject was born and read out a story that has some relevance. You could enlarge a photocopy and display it while you speak.

Original back issues of most of the main national and regional newspapers (subject to availability) can be bought from Historic Newspapers. They stock papers going back to the 1800s, although some of the more popular dates may have sold out. Contact them on 01988 402221.

Or you could discover the events that happened on the day she or he was born, and tie them in to the subject's life. Someone with a shared birthday might also be amusing. You can do the same thing with the date of the wedding: someone famous might have been married on the same day, or a great war might have been declared! Think around the events for relevant jokes.

The History Channel's website includes a search facility for important events that took place on any date of the year. Check it out at www.historychannel.com

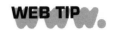

TODAY'S NEWS

Take a look through the newspapers and see if you can adapt any current stories to your speech. If you have access to a scanner and PC, you could even make authentic-looking changes to the piece.

You might want to put copies of any photographs, cuttings and other documents into a special book, which you could present to the couple as a further memento of the big day.

STAR-CROSS'D LOVERS

Look up the couple's star signs and see if they are supposed to be well matched. Reading out the characteristics of the signs can also lead to laughs, whether through spooky accuracy or, more realistically, amusing mismatches. Adapt, add bits or even make them up if it makes them funnier.

You could also read a prediction for that star sign from the day's newspapers – if they're not funny, relevant or irrelevant enough, make them up. 'A quiet day for Librans [or whatever]' should raise a chuckle. You could even try numerology (where birth-dates and names have numerical meanings) or find out which of the Chinese animal signs the subject was born under.

A ROSE BY ANY OTHER NAME

Grab a name dictionary and look up the meanings of the couple's names. You might come up with something funny or relevant. Surnames can also be researched – and these might be particularly appropriate if the bride is to take the groom's name.

I looked up the names of some couples I know and came up with the following:

A 'victory' together with a 'handsome at birth'.

A pair whose first names are both actually Scottish surnames – neither of whom have anything to do with Scotland. And his surname means 'descendant of a sea warrior'.

A 'fit to be loved' teamed up with a 'champion'.

One who is 'just', together with one who is 'snub-nosed' (he actually has got quite a pointy nose).

A girl who is 'lovable' together with a man who 'takes by the heel', i.e. a supplanter.

So a fair amount of ammunition for jokes, as well as opportunity to say something heartfelt, there.

JOKES

Obviously, telling jokes is a good way to enliven your speech. But there's nothing worse than a clumsy link to a joke that has nothing to do with the proceedings. Keep it topical or relevant.

SUGGESTED INTRODUCTIONS

I don't know the details of your wedding or the people concerned and it's vitally important to make your speech personal. If you've familiarised yourself with the particular jobs assigned to your role, and you've done your research, most of the work has already been done.

>> p31

How to start?

But that's no help when you're sitting staring at a blank sheet of paper, with an equally blank mind. Looking at this book's main section on openings (in chapter 3) should give you some hints and tips about how to make an attention-grabbing opening. If you're *still* stumped, here are a few suggestions to get you started:

FATHER OF THE BRIDE

'Ladies and gentlemen, attending my daughter's wedding today has taken me on a mental journey back – how many years?! – to my own wedding ...'

'Today is Janet and John's big day – and they've dropped a big hint that it will be an even better day if I keep my speech short, so you can all get to the bar. But it's not every day a father gives his daughter away, so I will ask for just a few minutes of your time ...'

'I had thought I might be nervous about standing up here and speaking to you all, but it's been such a wonderful day, and I'm so proud of Janet, that the nerves have just disappeared.'

'Every father looks forward with a mixture of pride and trepidation to the day when he is called upon to give his daughter away in marriage. Having been through it today I certainly feel very proud. And the only trepidation is about how I'm going to pay for this lot!'

'What a day! It's been such a pleasure to give my daughter away. My only regret is that I didn't do it years ago …'

(WHEN THE MOTHER OF THE BRIDE IS DEAD) 'The bride's father traditionally speaks both for himself and on behalf of the bride's mother. Sadly, my wife is no longer with us but, if she was, I know she would be as happy and proud as I am to see Janet and John getting married today.'

(WHEN THE BRIDE HAS BEEN MARRIED BEFORE) 'When Janet and John came to see us to tell us they were getting married, I was delighted. As you know, Janet has been married before. I'm glad that experience hasn't put her off a second try. But, Janet, if you ever think of trying for a third time, don't come to me for help!'

(WHEN BOTH HAVE BEEN MARRIED BEFORE) 'Ladies and gentlemen, all marriages are special. But second ones are doubly so, because it is a time for renewed hope.'

GROOM

'Ladies and gentlemen, my wife and I would like to start by saying thank you, James, for those kind words and good wishes.'

'My wife and I would like to say thank you to you all for coming to help us celebrate our wedding today. It's been a fantastic day, thanks to my wonderful wife and to the power of Imodium, without which I wouldn't be here today.'

'Today really has been the happiest day of my life. I've had quite a good life up to now and so that's quite an achievement. The only events that have come close for me were when Chelsea won the FA Cup and when I won the junior boys' egg and spoon race.'

'When I first saw my wife, I wasted no time in going over to chat her up. But that was mainly because my mate said he was going to if I didn't. Well, I'm glad I beat him to it because that evening was the beginning of a wonderful love story.'

(WHEN THEY HAVE LIVED TOGETHER FOR A LONG TIME) 'A few people have asked me why we're bothering to get married after all these years. The answer is that I wanted to stand up in public and let the world know how much Janet means to me. We've been happy together for a long time, but we felt it was time to move our relationship on and make a public commitment.'

'I know Janet and I have spent a while getting round to our wedding day. It's not that we weren't sure about each other. We were just giving James a chance to save up!'

(WHEN HE HAS BEEN MARRIED BEFORE) 'There's a first time for everything – and sometimes a second.'

(WHEN THERE ARE CHILDREN INVOLVED) 'This is a very big day for Janet and myself, but it's also a big day for Janet's children, Rod, Jane and Freddie. And my first thank you is to them, for welcoming me into their family. I know that they mean the world to Janet and I know I'm very lucky to be a part of their lives.'

BEST MAN

'First of all, on behalf of the bridesmaids, I'd like to thank John for his kind words. It's traditional for the best man to compliment the bridesmaids and, on this occasion, that's certainly an easy task – don't they look lovely?'

'I'd like to share with you today some very special words I overheard while the wedding photographs were being taken. I'm sorry I don't know the names of the guests concerned, but I thought I should pass on what they said. One of the ladies confided in the other that she hadn't seen her husband for 20 years: "He went out to buy a cabbage and never came back." The other looked shocked and said: "What on earth did you do?" "Oh," said the first, "I just opened a tin of peas."'

'I'm sure you've all heard stories about people getting cold feet before a wedding – and I've got to tell you, up until this moment I wasn't sure I was actually going to make it.'

'Unaccustomed as I am to pubic spanking ... er, I mean ...'

'I knew early on in their relationship that John was truly in love – and not just because he started missing nights out with the lads and buying better clothes. No, I could tell by the way he looked at Janet, and I had no trouble recognising that she was the one for him.'

'It's not often that us blokes get to talk about love. But I'm delighted that I've had the opportunity to do so today. And if there are any single women among the guests, who feel touched by my sensitivity, I'll be at the bar later.'

BRIDE

'Most of you know me well. And most of you will therefore not be surprised that we've decided to break with tradition and allow the blushing bride to say a few words.'

'Surely you didn't think I was going to sit there and let John speak for me … I never have in the past!'

'Some of you might think it's a bit forward for a bride to get up and make a speech. Well, wait till I tell you how I proposed …'

'I couldn't resist this opportunity to embarrass my new husband in public. And probably not for the last time.'

(WHEN SHE HAS BEEN MARRIED BEFORE) 'Most of you know that this is the second time I've been a bride. I thought the first time was for life but that didn't work out. Still, the nature of mistakes is that we learn from them and I know that my marriage to John is going to be very different and I'm confident that this is my last time in the white dress.'

(WHEN THERE ARE CHILDREN INVOLVED) See groom (p.154).

SON STANDING IN FOR FATHER OF THE BRIDE
'"Our father, who art in heaven …" Well, mine is, and that's why I'm standing in for him today …'

SOMEONE ELSE STANDING IN FOR FATHER OF THE BRIDE
'When Mary asked me to stand in and make the speech usually performed by the father of the bride, I was very touched. I have spent a long time thinking about what my dear brother/friend would have liked to say on this occasion and one thing I do know is that he would have been very proud.'

'When I was small, my brother James was always getting me into trouble – and now look at the mess he's got me into! I'm sure he's looking down and laughing at my awkward attempts at speech-making.'

'Many of you will not know me, so I'd like to begin by introducing myself.'

STAND-IN FOR FATHER OF THE BRIDE/BEST MAN WHO'S ILL
'I know I'm probably not the person most of you expected to be speaking at this point, but Jim is unfortunately too ill to make it today. I spoke to him this morning though and he's promised me that he'll be scrutinising the video to see if I was an adequate stand-in. Jim

asked me to send his apologies and best wishes to Janet and John, and I'm sure you all join me in wishing him a speedy recovery and hoping that he can soon get right back on his hang-glider!'

MOTHER OF THE BRIDE

'If my husband was still alive, I know he'd say, "Mary, you never *could* keep quiet!" But I think I'm entitled to say a few words today of all days. Janet was very close to her father and they are so alike in so many ways. But today is a happy occasion and so we're going to look to the future and not dwell on the past.'

WHEN SOMEONE CLOSE TO THE COUPLE HAS DIED RECENTLY

'For many of us, there is a little sadness mixed in with today's joy. And that's because of the recent loss of Jim. Those of us who knew him find it hard to believe that he's not among us today and we would like to pay tribute to him and say thank you for his life.

'But today is Janet and John's wedding day and I know Jim wouldn't want us to dwell on sad thoughts.'

IF THE STAND-IN IS THERE FOR A HAPPIER REASON

'Many of you will be surprised to see me standing here today in Steve's place. And believe me, 24 hours ago I thought I was going to be sitting around and knocking back the champagne with the rest of you.

'But John called me and told me something that Steve's girlfriends could have told me years ago – that he was unable to perform on the big occasion.'

As for finding jokes, the field is enormous. Rent out comedy videos and films, look up gags on the Net, note down funnies in papers and mags. There are plenty of wedding-joke books around, too. Ask people for their favourite joke. But remember, very often, your own raw original material will be much funnier than any stuff that's borrowed.

TOASTS

Most of the wedding speeches traditionally include a toast, and the English custom is usually to keep it simple and announce, 'To the bride and groom!' or 'To the bridesmaids'.

But you can make the occasion very special by choosing a longer toast. You may even ask someone else to propose it – particularly useful if you have other close friends or family who would not otherwise have a role to play.

Here are a few suggestions:

- May your home always be too small to hold all of your friends;

  May you both live as long as you want and never want as long as you live;

  May your troubles be less and your blessings be more,
  And nothing but happiness come through your door.

- May your love always last and your happiness always be assured.

- May the happiest day of your past be the saddest day of your future;

  May you love each other more than yesterday but less than tomorrow;

  May the love you share for ever remain as beautiful as the bride looks today;

  May your wishes always come true and may you always get more than you wish for;

  May your hands be forever joined in friendship and your hearts forever joined in love;

  May you live as long as you want to and want to as long as you live;

  May your love be modern enough to survive the times and old-fashioned enough to last for ever;

  May you live long, laugh often, and love much;

  May the love you feel today be present always, for ever and a day.

- It is said when a child finds true love the parents find true joy.

- May the most you ever wish for be the least you receive.

- They say you get married for better or worse.
  May your lives together be far better than worse.

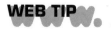 **WEB TIP**

Find more toasts at weddings.about.com/style/weddings/. If you really get a kick out of this – and public speaking in general – why not check out Toastmasters International at www.toastmasters.org.uk.

READINGS

Another way of involving close friends and family in your wedding is to ask them to perform a reading, whether you're getting married in church or in a civil ceremony.

If you've been asked to do a reading, I'm sure you've taken the invitation as a huge compliment, but you're probably still very nervous about the prospect – especially if you are going to have to read from the Bible. And in church too! Poems also fill many people with terror, as they wrestle with the short lines and unfamiliar punctuation.

Well, fear not, my friend. Help is at hand. Read on …

It's a great honour to be asked to read at someone's wedding – but it can be scary too.

CHOOSING A READING

Sometimes kind couples will simply give you a book, tell you which page you're reading and send you off to practise.

However, others will ask you to choose – either because they can't be bothered, or because you appear to have – or claim to have – some kind of literary expertise.

IN CHURCH If the wedding is taking place in church, the vicar will normally be able to supply a selection of suitable biblical passages.

Read them through, and really consider which one is most appropriate for the couple who are getting married (not which one is the shortest, or has the least big words).

I have provided the references for some of the most popular biblical passages below, but once you've chosen, just run it past the vicar or priest for approval – it is their church, after all.

Many vicars will also allow you to read a secular text, but here things might get a bit more tricky. Your average priest or vicar is likely to give the thumbs up to the old classics – Shakespeare, Wordsworth; that kind of thing. But they may be suspicious of anything they're unfamiliar with or suspect of being too modern and trendy.

However, some vicars might be much more open-minded or open to persuasion. They may even welcome new sources into their churches.

A CIVIL CEREMONY Don't imagine that just because you're *not* in a church that anything goes. Far from it.

The first and most important thing to remember is that civil ceremonies – whether in a State-licensed venue or in a Register Office – do not allow readings with any religious content at all. It's obvious that this means no Bible readings, prayers or hymns, but it also applies to other 'spiritual' poems, such as the ever-popular 'Desiderata' ('Go placidly amid the noise and haste').

Just like the readings in the vicar's church, you must clear any reading with the registrar, or whoever is conducting the ceremony.

The vicar and registrar are only one part of the equation though. You also need to choose something that's appropriate for the couple themselves.

Humanist weddings, or other alternative ceremonies, allow total freedom and may be worth considering if you're set on pieces that the church/Registrar won't approve of.

If you're choosing a non-religious reading, where on earth do you start?

If you're choosing for your own wedding, the following suggestions might help. If you're choosing the reading for a friend, you might want to go through it with them:

Do you have a favourite poet/author/book that might be appropriate?

Look in books of quotations under sections such as 'love' and 'marriage'. Note any particular quotations or authors that you find appealing and look into them more carefully.

There are several books of love poetry or suggested readings. Invest in one or see if your library can get it for you.

The British Humanist Association publishes a guide to non-religious wedding ceremonies, 'Sharing the Future', which includes a section on readings.

Contact them via www.humanism.org.uk, **or call 020 7430 0908.**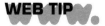

READINGS

Some suggested readings (I have left it to you to look them up):

Matthew 19:3–6

John 15:9-13 'Song of Songs' 2:13–14, 16; 8:6–7

Colossians 3:12–15

Genesis 2:18–24

Proverbs 5:15–19; 18:22

Ecclesiastes 4:9–12

Matthew 19:5–6

Mark 10:6–9

John 2:1–11

I Corinthians 7

RELIGIOUS READINGS If you're not very familiar with the Bible, it might seem daunting to have to choose a reading for your wedding. But the Bible really isn't difficult to read – you just need to take time.

Some families have traditional readings, which are used at all family weddings. Even if yours doesn't, you might want to ask your parents what was read at their wedding. Or if you've been asked to give a reading, you might want to choose one that was read at your own wedding, or at *your* parents' wedding. Although you won't mention that in church, you might want to explain to the couple, or the other guests, the reason behind your choice.

You also need to decide which version of the Bible you want to use. There is only one Bible, but there are a number of different versions, or translations. Your priest or vicar may have strong feelings about which you use, or may be happy for you to have the one you prefer. It's another thing that you should discuss with them in advance.

The King James's Bible is the old one, dating back to the 17th century. While some welcome it for its familarity and rich old-fashioned language, others find it out of date and difficult to understand.

There are several more modern versions – from the Revised Standard Version (RSV), which updates the traditional translations, to those like the New English Bible (NEB) or the Good News Bible, which try to be ultra-modern, replacing all the words that are no longer in common use.

Roman Catholics usually use the Jerusalem Bible, but that too is available in a newer version.

Compare these versions of I Corinthians 13:4–7 (which I chose for my own wedding, incidentally) – the first from the King James and the second from the NEB.

> 'Charity suffereth long, and is kind; charity envieth not; charity vaunteth not itself, is not puffed up, doth not behave itself unseemly, seeketh not her own, is not easily provoked, thinketh no evil; rejoiceth not in iniquity, but rejoiceth in the truth; beareth all things, believeth all things, hopeth all things, endureth all things.'

> 'Love is patient; love is kind and envies no one. Love is never boastful, nor conceited, nor rude; never selfish, nor quick to take offence. Love keeps no score of wrongs; does not gloat over other men's sins, but delights in the truth. There is nothing love cannot face; there is no limit to its faith, its hope, and its endurance.'

The Bible is divided into the Old and New Testaments and then further into a series of Books. Each Book divides into chapters, which divide further into verses. Quotations are identified first by the name of the book. After the name of the book comes the chapter number. Finally, there are the verse numbers.

Several of the books have commonly abbreviated titles. If you're not sure what you're looking for, there should be a table at the beginning of your Bible, listing all the abbreviations. It will also tell you the order of the books, so you can find them faster.

NON-RELIGIOUS READINGS Love poems are the most popular choice but poetry is such a personal thing that it's hard to narrow this down to a few suggestions. If you don't have a favourite poem or poet, you might like to start by looking at some of the following:

The Passionate Shepherd to his Love – Christopher Marlowe
Come live with me and be my Love,
And we will all the pleasures prove

My Love is Like a Red, Red Rose – Robert Burns
My love is like a red, red rose
That's newly sprung in June

A Dedication to My Wife – T S Eliot
To whom I owe the leaping delight
That quickens my senses in our wakingtime
And the rhythm that governs the repose of our sleepingtime,
The breathing in unison

If Thou Must Love Me – Elizabeth Barrett Browning
If thou must love me, let it be for naught
Except for love's sake only

CHECKLIST

Checklist for choosing a reading:

Has the reading been approved by the vicar/priest/registrar? ❏

Is it suitable? ❏

Is it about marriage, rather than just falling in love, or lust? ❏

Does the piece make sense as a piece of writing, without
　　needing any further explanation? ❏

Does it fit in with the prayers, other readings and hymns? ❏

Are you sure it won't offend anyone? ❏

Is it the right length – not too short and not too long? ❏

Does the reader feel comfortable with it? ❏

The Bargain – Sir Philip Sidney

My true love hath my heart, and I have his

There are dozens of suggestions for readings on the internet. You might like to try:

www.speeches.com

Weddings.about.com/style/weddings

www.lovepoetry.com

www.weddingguide.co.uk

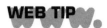
WEB TIP

SUMMARY

Rules are there to be broken – but you can only break the rules if you know what they are in the first place. You now know why traditions exist and when it's OK to change them. You should also be more inspired about choosing an appropriate reading. Let's recap:

Work out who should speak and what they should say

Stick to tradition or adapt it to your special needs – but make sure everyone's clear about their role.

Step-families, bereavement and other tricky matters

Be sensible and sensitive and no one will get hurt.

Research

Use the insider tips on research specific to wedding speeches.

Suggested intros

Getting started is often the hardest bit. Use these suggestions as a way to get going … then it's up to you.

Toasts

Think about this charming, but neglected tradition

Readings

Offer the right passage to the right people at the right ceremony. These suggestions should give you some inspiration and help you find your way round the Bible.

10

SPEAKING TO

THE MEDIA

* FEAR OF THE PRESS

* PRESS RELEASES

* APPROACHING THE MEDIA

* EXCLUSIVES – KISS & TELLS

* HOW TO HANDLE THAT PHONE CALL

* SIMPLE DOS & DON'TS

* MAKING THE MOST OF YOUR MEDIA TIME

* DEALING WITH DIFFICULT QUESTIONS

* EMERGENCIES & INCIDENTS

It's ironic, but the press gets a very bad press. There are several reasons why you might find yourself at the sharp end of a journalist's pencil; or the fluffy end of a radio mike; or the wide end of a TV camera.

If you're running a campaign, you might want to use the media to publicise your cause. You might want to get some editorial coverage to help boost your business. You might witness a major accident (God forbid) or be involved in a dramatic rescue. You might find that the spotty oik you used to date in the fifth form has now become the latest rock god. You might even get off with someone famous and decide to pose half-naked and sell your kiss and tell to the *News of the World*.

Whether your motives are altruistic or purely for financial gain, it's probably only a matter of time before you get your Andy Warhol 15 minutes of fame. Much of this section deals with issues you might not traditionally regard as public speaking – but in fact, speaking to the media is likely to reach a bigger audience than any conference centre or village hall. Also, you'll find lots of tips on writing press releases and other ways of attracting the media's attention.

Of course, this doesn't necessarily involve speaking, but unless you know how to get onto the news agenda, you'll never get the chance.

FEAR OF THE PRESS

You can hardly open a magazine now, or turn on the television, without some bleeding-heart celebrity complaining about press intrusion. The tragic death of Princess Diana also served to further blacken the name of the British newspaper industry. Much of the criticism has been well deserved and the crisis has made editors think twice about issues of intrusion and harassment.

However, a drawback of the negative coverage has been that ordinary people are often terrified of the press, fearing that their names will be dragged through the dirt; that they will be misquoted and misunderstood; or that they will be ridiculed. I must emphasise that this is *not* the case.

In the first place, you're not a celebrity. It's highly unlikely that anyone is going to go through your bins or try to trip you up into talking about something you would rather have kept quiet. Journalists are in the business of selling newspapers, it's true. And celebrity scoops certainly have a big part to play in selling newspapers. But readers also love good luck stories, amusing anecdotes, tales of the triumph of ordinary people, and they adore the idea of people pulling together for a common cause.

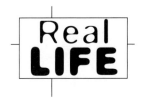

Look at the petrol crisis of summer 2000 – the press had a field day with the idea of people power. Ordinary truckers and farmers found themselves leading a national campaign that affected almost every area of British life and dominated the front pages for days on end. Those ordinary truckers and farmers had the chance to put their views across when they were interviewed by journalists. And the journalists were

happy to reflect the nation's views and give voice to the protesters.

Look too at the campaigns to find organ transplants for children. Here we have ordinary parents who found themselves in the extraordinary situation of having to fight for their child's life. By going to the media with their plea, the search for a suitable donor instantly becomes national or world-wide. Countless lives have been saved, thanks to such campaigns.

There are literally thousands and thousands of such examples – the local press in particular is constantly running various campaigns on behalf of local people.

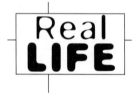

When I was a cub reporter on a local newspaper, I launched a number of campaigns on issues affecting the town where I worked. But one of the stories I'm proudest of only affected a single family. A local woman had travelled to America on holiday but while there she had suffered a sudden and serious heart attack. Luckily, she had medical insurance and was able to secure the best hospital treatment. But she was so ill that doctors advised her husband to call their daughters to warn them that their mother was probably going to die any day. Amazingly, she pulled through and was able to fly home again in a matter of weeks. But on returning to the UK, she faced horrendous bills from all sides. Her husband had returned the hire car a day late and had been charged a hefty penalty fee. A credit card that had been used to make all those pricey transatlantic phone calls was demanding immediate payment because the charges were sky-high. Her husband had had to stay somewhere near the hospital. This sick woman was at her wits' end when she turned up in our newspaper office, begging for any help we could lend. I must admit, I was sceptical – we were only a tiny local paper, with none of the sway held by the nationals. But by the end of the day, I had halved the bills. The credit card company waived some of the charges and agreed to take the rest of the payment in affordable monthly sums. The car hire company scrapped the penalty fee. We ran the story as the front page splash and various local organisations rushed to help. Not only were the financial headaches solved, but the woman in question was inundated with offers of help in other ways.

If one story, in one small provincial newspaper, can do all that in one day, imagine what you can achieve for your campaign if you harness the power of the press.

OK, JOURNALISTS ARE OBVIOUSLY THE MOST WONDERFUL PEOPLE ON THE PLANET – WHAT NOW? Well, having allayed your worst fears, I would temper my advice with a few stern words of caution. You can get what you want from the press if you've got something to say, you find the right people to say it to and you play it straight.

Let's go through the process and we'll find the most important dos and don'ts along the way.

The first thing you need to do is to think about whether anyone really cares about what you want to say. You need to present your story in the most newsworthy way, by thinking like an editor.

CHECKLIST

Run through the following checklist and see if you can say yes to any of the questions:

	yes	no
Is the subject already recognised as an issue?	❏	❏
Is there anyone famous involved?	❏	❏
Is there a famous organisation involved?	❏	❏
Is the issue fashionable, topical or current?	❏	❏
Is the subject an event or problem that's happening right now?	❏	❏
Will the subject have a significant impact?	❏	❏
Will the impact be felt directly by people? Or groups of people?	❏	❏
Will the impact be felt locally? Or globally?	❏	❏

---

	yes	no
Is there a real power-struggle involved? Does it involve individuals fighting against a major organisation?	❏	❏
Do you simply have a good story to tell?	❏	❏
Does the story involve children? Or animals? Or old people? Or sick people? Or anyone else who might grab the public imagination?	❏	❏
Does the story have an emotional impact on those who hear it?	❏	❏
Does the story or issue have a visual side? Are there photo opportunities? Might there be an opportunity to film something dramatic?	❏	❏
Does the story fit in to a theme that always interests people, e.g. the triumph of love over circumstances; a dramatic rescue; a community who pulled together where others might have fallen apart; a local boy who saw an opportunity and pursued it to impressive ends; racism; sexism, etc.?	❏	❏
Is there anything funny about it?	❏	❏
Is there anything innovative about it?	❏	❏
Is there anything really big about it?	❏	❏
Is it a 'first' in any way?	❏	❏
Is there anything wacky about it?	❏	❏

	yes	no
Does it touch on issues that might be relevant to a large number of people? If they heard your story could it help them improve their life/health/understanding/consumer rights?	❏	❏
Have you organised an event that's open to the public?	❏	❏
Have you won an award, been appointed to an important organisation or otherwise achieved recognition for what you do?	❏	❏
Have you published a book or CD? Have you mounted an exhibition?	❏	❏
Have you provided some kind of important service to your community?	❏	❏
Are you standing for some kind of public office or important role?	❏	❏
Are you involved in a major investigation, inquiry or court case?	❏	❏
Are you offering a totally new product or service?	❏	❏
Are you looking for volunteers?	❏	❏
Are you offering training or apprenticeships?	❏	❏
Have you won the lottery? Or a lot of money/big prize in another competition?	❏	❏
Are you about to appear on television?	❏	❏
Are you offering franchises of your business?	❏	❏

	yes	no
Have you opened a new branch of your business? Or moved your headquarters somewhere else?	❏	❏
Have you received an impressive qualification? Has a member of your staff?	❏	❏
Are you throwing your office/factory open to visitors for a day?	❏	❏
Are you having a general meeting?	❏	❏
Has your company sponsored a major event?	❏	❏

If you can say 'yes' to any of those questions, you've probably got a story. The more positive answers, the better the story.

If you didn't shout 'yes' many times, that list itself should help you think of ways you could add news value to your campaign.

But there are lots of things you can do to boost the story's newsworthiness. Journalists talk about a story being 'sexy', or saying it's 'got legs', by which they mean it's a good, exciting story.

If you only answered 'yes' to the rather dull questions – 'Are you offering training?', 'Are you standing for office?' or some of the other questions towards the bottom of the list – you might need to make your story a bit more sexy.

If you are staging an event, or you run an attraction, or the like, don't forget to offer the journalist a free press ticket, or two if you can afford it. It'll be worth it in the long run.

MAKING IT SEXIER
Here are a few ideas:

1 Do a survey – especially in the 'silly season' of August, when news runs dry and journalists are desperate to fill the pages.

2 Get someone to turn it into a report – another goodie for August. Persuade a charity or educational organisation to lend their support to your report.

3 Hold a vote or election of some kind.

4 Announce an appointment.

5 Make it topical: look for an angle that chimes with something else that's happening in the news.

6 Hire a PR (this will cost money but might be worth considering).

7 Approach a publication or programme about mounting a joint event or joining in with their existing ones.

8 Approach a publication or programme about the possibility of them sponsoring your event. You'll get money AND publicity!

9 Tie it in with an anniversary.

10 Issue a set of guidelines, or a handy guide or a set of facts.

11 Wait for a relevant time of year and tie the campaign to it: parents will be more receptive about campaigns to teach children to swim during the summer; they'll be more sympathetic to the plight of the homeless during the winter.

12 Wait for a relevant date and tie the campaign to it: fertility and egg donation at Easter, perhaps; or a campaign for a maternity ward at Christmas.

13 Get someone famous involved.

14 Do something controversial.

15 Stage an event.

16 Get lots of people involved and announce their names. Take the journalists on a trip or outing – it must be something they'll really want to go on, though, and they must be sure they'll get a story out of it.

17 Create a competition or set of awards.

18 Form a delegation to approach the government, council or other relevant body.

19 Stage a sit-in, a blockade or other form of protest.

20 Stage a concert.

21 Organise a march.

22 Call for a boycott.

23 Write a letter to someone newsworthy or publish a letter from someone newsworthy or about something newsworthy.

24 Create a 'day' – like Red Nose Day, Jeans for Genes day – there are hundreds of these!

25 If you don't want to invite the media to an event, for any reason – or if they can't come – why not videotape the event yourself. If the event ends up in the headlines, they might use your footage.

I mentioned the 'silly season' above. If you're not sure how truly newsworthy your story is, why not wait until August. All the traditional sources of news are on holiday and stories are woefully thin on the ground. Editors will greet your story with heartfelt joy.

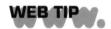 **lamar.colostate.edu/~hallahan/hpubty has lots more ideas about how to get publicity.**

You might start the ball rolling on your media campaign with a simple phone call to the right journalist, but you could – especially if you want to reach more than one publication – send out a press release.

PRESS RELEASES

I know what you're thinking. Aren't we straying off the point somewhat? This is a public speaking book. Press releases have nothing to do with public speaking. Right?

Right. But if you don't grab the attention of the journalists you're trying to reach, they won't be asking you to speak at all.

You've already decided what your story is, and you've thought of everything you can to make that story more sexy. But you still need to hone your approach.

 DON'T dilute your message. If you have several angles to your story, don't confuse the media by trying to shoe-horn them all into the same press release.

 DO decide what your overall message is, and stick to this for the first release.

Let's look at a fictitious example:

Seven-year-old Kerry Potts is disabled and the authorities said she couldn't go to the local school unless it had proper wheelchair access. The authority decided not to fund the alterations and told Kerry she would have to go to a school in the city centre. Her neighbour, Angela Smith, was so upset that she decided to start a fund-raising campaign.

She discussed the idea with friends and neighbours, who were very supportive. Their first idea was to do a sponsored head shave in the school hall, to help raise the money. One of them knew a local celebrity and agreed to approach him about getting involved. Another runs a local business and his staff offered to put on a barn-dance in the school gymnasium, as part of the fund-raising. At this point, Mrs Smith decided to call the local newspaper to tell them what was going on.

Let's examine how she managed the events to get maximum coverage.

Giving the press everything in one go could well get you a story – but only one story and a slightly muddled one at that.

Angela decided to break it down into several bits and do a new press release each week. She hoped this approach meant the story would be in the paper every week. The stories themselves were a little smaller but she won the support of the paper, who placed them in prominent positions on their pages.

The stories broke down roughly like this:

WEEK ONE Little Kerry is banned from village school – neighbours start fund-raising campaign.

WEEK TWO Villagers pledge to go bald to help little Kerry.

WEEK THREE Workers stage barn-dance to help little Kerry.

WEEK FOUR (having had the definite go-ahead from the celebrity) – Local star John Morton joins fight for little Kerry and wields clippers in sponsored head shave.

WEEK FIVE Morton opens garden for village party in little Kerry campaign.

Well, you get the drift. To try to put all those things into one press release would have been confusing.

PLUS a 'drip-drip' approach, with a story each week, kept Angela's

TIP
Keep your release simple and avoid hype. Remember, thousands of press releases pour into newspaper offices. Journalists don't need whizzes and bangs to make them notice yours – if you've got a good story and you tell it clearly, they'll notice. Follow our template for a good press release (see over).

Sums the story up in as few words as possible

PRESS RELEASE TEMPLATE

1. DATE

2. HEADLINE
Villagers start campaign for little Kerry to attend local school.

3. SUBHEAD
Authorities rule that 7-year-old disabled child must travel to Donchester for education – but local people pledge to raise cash to equip the village school.

Slightly longer – expands on headline

Opens the story – keep it short

4. INTRO
Little Marching residents have launched a fund-raising campaign, after education authorities ruled that wheelchair user Kerry Potts must attend school in Donchester city centre, twelve miles from her home.

5. SECOND PARAGRAPH
The villagers decided on the action after a shock ruling that Little Marching School will not receive the government funding necessary to adapt it for wheelchair access.

Together with intro, these two paragraphs should tell the who, what, why, when, how

Sums up the situation in the words of someone involved

6. KEY QUOTE
Kerry's mother, Tanya Potts, said: 'Kerry has grown up in the village and all her friends are here. We are supporters of the local school and we don't want to send her to a much bigger school in the city centre. I'm bitterly disappointed that the authorities won't find the money to pay for the adaptations.'

Keep it brief, but simply tell the story in chronological order

7. TELL THE STORY
Mr and Mrs Potts put Kerry's name down for the local school in April, but they were told that her disability meant the building would have to be assessed for wheelchair access.

The authorities ruled that the school was not

suitable, but the work necessary was assessed and applications were made for funding.

But at a meeting on Monday, the Potts heard the application had been turned down and Kerry would have to attend the nearest suitable school, Donchester City School.

8. SECOND OR MORE QUOTES

Mrs Potts added: 'Donchester City School is twelve miles from our home and it's an hour's journey, there and back. Kerry might be disabled but she shouldn't be made to feel different to the other children. She should be educated here, among her friends.'

As you tell the story, you may want to include more quotes to illustrate it and vary the pace of the release

9. BACK TO THE STORY

The Pottses' neighbour, Mrs Angela Smith, decided to mount a campaign to raise the £5,000 needed to pay for the changes.

Return to the main story

10. INCLUDE ALL THE DETAILS THE PUBLIC WILL NEED TO KNOW

Local people have been invited to attend a meeting at Little Marching School hall on Tuesday 19 May at 7 pm.

Mrs Smith said: 'We're asking everyone in the village to come, so that we can put our heads together and come up with some ways to raise this money for Kerry.'

Details for people who might get involved

11. INCLUDE ALL THE DETAILS THE JOURNALISTS WILL NEED TO KNOW

Contact:

Mrs Tanya Potts – 01222 839567

Mrs Angela Smith – 01222 839574

Details for the press to follow up on

12. NOTE TO EDITOR

Kerry suffers from spina bifida and has been unable to walk since birth.

Optional: any background information that might not be suitable as part of the release, but would be useful

PRESS RELEASE

VILLAGERS CAMPAIGN FOR GIRL TO ATTEND LOCAL SCHOOL

Authorities rule that seven-year-old disabled child must travel to Donchester for education – but local people pledge to raise cash to equip the village school

Little Marching residents have launched a fund-raising campaign, after education authorities ruled that wheelchair user Kerry Potts must attend school in Donchester city centre, twelve miles from her home.

The villagers decided on the action after a shock ruling that Little Marching School will not receive the government funding necessary to adapt it for wheelchair access.

Kerry's mother, Tanya Potts, said: 'Kerry has grown up in the village and all her friends are here. We are supporters of the local school and we don't want to send her to a much bigger school in the city centre. I'm bitterly disappointed that the authorities won't find the money to pay for the adaptations.'

Mr and Mrs Potts put Kerry's name down for the local school in April, but they were told that her disability meant the building would have to be assessed for wheelchair access.

The authorities ruled that the school was not suitable, but the work necessary was assessed and applications were made for funding.

But at a meeting on Monday, the Pottses heard the application had been turned down and Kerry would have to attend the nearest suitable school, Donchester City School.

Mrs Potts added: 'Donchester City School is twelve miles from our home and it's an hour's journey, there and back. Kerry might be disabled but

ILLUSTRATION 18:   A finished press release should look something like this – but fit it on one page!

she shouldn't be made to feel different to the other children. She should be educated here, among her friends.'

The Pottses' neighbour, Mrs Angela Smith, decided to mount a campaign to raise the £5,000 needed to pay for the changes.

Local people have been invited to attend a meeting at Little Marching School hall on Tuesday 19 May at 7 pm.

Mrs Smith said: 'We're asking everyone in the village to come, so that we can put our heads together and come up with some ways to raise this money for Kerry.'

Ends

Contact:

Mrs Tanya Potts – 01222 839567

Mrs Angela Smith – 01222 839574

Note to editors: Kerry suffers from spina bifida and has been unable to walk since birth.

campaign in people's minds for longer.

When writing or speaking about dates for important events, don't just say '19 May', say 'Tuesday 19 May' – it will help people to remember it.

DON'T go into a long-winded history of everything you've ever done. Try to edit it down to a few words: Clothing manufacturer N Brown and Sons, which specialises in dancewear ...

DON'T write more than a single page of A4, if you can possibly help it.

DON'T try to sell your product. Keep that approach for your clients. When talking to journalists, simply provide information about it.

DON'T use long words or jargon. Newspapers don't so why should you?

DON'T try to flog them a story that's way out of date. If it happened months ago, sorry, you've missed the boat and you'll have to come up with something new.

DON'T exaggerate or hype.

DO print your release on a computer, or at least a very good typewriter. Borrow one if necessary – but NEVER hand-write releases. No one will take you seriously.

DO keep the release brief but include all the necessary background information. If you're writing about a complicated issue, the journalists will be grateful for the explanation.

DO offer to give them more information, if necessary. You might want to simplify the issue – let the editor decide exactly which areas they want to explore further.

DO explain what your company does, if you're writing about a business issue.

JARGONBUSTER!

Embargo: a request for a publication to wait until a certain date before publishing the story.

DO include additional information on a separate sheet if you feel you need to say more. Draw up a company biog on to a separate sheet of A4.

DO check, check and double check your spelling.

DO avoid clichés.

DO get someone else to read the release before you send it out.

DON'T be too blatantly promotional – too false. Editors are happy to carry news, but they don't like being over-manipulated by someone trying to get a slice of the action. Make your story news, real news.

CHECKLIST FOR NEW RELEASES

Have you included:

date that you're sending the release? ❏

embargo date – if appropriate? ❏

contact name and phone number (during office hours)? ❏

headline? ❏

subhead? ❏

intro? ❏

key quote? ❏

story? ❏

all relevant dates in full (including day of the week)? ❏

all relevant times? ❏

all relevant addresses (with details of how to get there, if necessary)? ❏

full names (spelt correctly)? ❏

any background information? ❏

APPROACHING THE MEDIA

Firstly, you need to appreciate that you might get very little coverage, or even none at all. Don't be disheartened. Even the act of sending the release has made that one journalist aware of you.

But you don't want to be constantly sending releases to the wrong people. Not only is it a waste of your time and money, but any journalist finding an irrelevant release on their cluttered desk will become irritated and will throw it away. At best, they'll forget about it. At worst, they'll remember your name and mentally give you a black mark.

But there are ways to make your releases more effective:

DO get the right target.

DO log on and have a good look round if you're targeting a website.

DO phone up and ask for the name and job title of the person you need to send it to if you're satisfied that they cover your kind of story. Most magazines carry names, job titles, direct lines and even email addresses for their key staff. Look it up. If you've hit the right target, they'll be delighted to hear from you.

DON'T grab some listing for 'magazines' and send out releases willy nilly.

DON'T just send your press release off to the BBC. Read your target publication and listen to or watch the programme.

GET THE NAME RIGHT

When you get that person's name do *double check* the spelling and job title. I know I've got an unusual name but when I was a journalist, I was so sick of people spelling my name wrong that I often chucked away releases with barely a glance if they'd got it wrong.

Never, ever, abbreviate anyone's name without asking them. It's not friendly, it's rude. If their listing says Charles, they're Charles to you. Not Charlie, not Chas, not Chuck. Charles.

GET THE TIMING RIGHT

Glossy magazines usually have long lead times – between two and four months. And special editions, such as a Christmas issue, might be planned out even earlier than that. So contacting them in April to say you've heard they're covering your subject in May isn't much good.

But if your product is going to be a secret until the last minute, trust the journalist. Most will be more than happy to sign embargos – meaning they can't breathe a word until a certain date – if it means they're going to get the scoop.

DON'T irritate them by refusing to tell them. How will they know how much space to plan for it unless they know the facts?

GET UP TO DATE

DON'T think that because someone gave you the name of the news editor in 1973, they're still there.

DO check out that staffing column I mentioned above.

GET ON THE RIGHT SIDE OF YOUR MEDIA CONTACT.

Many media guides tell you to follow up your press release with a call.

BE VERY CAREFUL WITH THIS. I used to be driven up the wall with irritating PRs – total strangers with whom I'd never done business before – phoning me up on a news day and asking me how I was. Then they plagued me by asking me if I'd received their fax. If you mailed it – they've got it. OK?

If you hear nothing and you're anxious, you can call a few days later. But be direct and to the point. Make it clear you're not hassling them.

WHAT ABOUT EMAILS?

Some journalists like to receive press releases by email – others don't. The best thing to do is to call and ask. If you do email your releases, remember:

DON'T send huge attachments that will take the journalist ages to download.

DON'T hound the journalist. If they don't reply to your email, take the hint and leave them alone.

DO make it clear that you can send pictures, products or other attachments, and ask the journalist to mail you back if they'd like to receive them.

DO be careful about 'netiquette'!

DO write the address of your website (the URL) if you have one. Most word-processing systems will turn this URL into a link, so

JARGONBUSTER!

Netiquette: from 'internet' and 'etiquette'. The correct form of behaviour to use while working on the internet.

the recipient can click on it and be connected directly to your website.

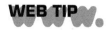

WEB TIP For more information about netiquette, including a quiz to test your expertise, visit www.albion.com/netiquette.

EXCLUSIVES – KISS & TELLS

If your story is particularly hot, you might want to offer it to a publication as an exclusive. Or a newspaper or magazine might take the initiative and ask you not to speak to anyone else about it.

You need to think carefully about exclusives – a newspaper might promise the earth, but exclusives can end up tripping you up. If you're out to make money, you'll need to sign exclusivity deals – no paper will pay you for your story unless they're the only one carrying the tale.

JARGONBUSTER!
Exclusive: strictly speaking, a story that is only told to one publication.

But if you're talking to the press for another reason – to publicise your business, for example – exclusives can be counter-productive. If rival newspapers feel they've missed out on a great story, they might be miffed enough to run a counter-story, attacking you or your business. At the very least, they'll be much more receptive to anyone else approaching them with a less than flattering angle.

Kiss and tell stories are almost always told on an exclusive basis. The teller (and indeed kisser) can often command a high price for their story – if it concerns the right celebrity. Anyone who's constantly in the newspapers is likely to be a lucrative target – but usually only if they're married. A romp with a young, free and single celebrity might earn you a few column inches, but it's rarely going to make you rich.

DO think deeply about your motives for telling your story about a celebrity, why you should tell it, and about how it would make you look in the eyes of the world.

You can also offer exclusives by genre – you might promise that you won't speak to any other national newspaper except the *Sun*, but you might also promise to tell your story to *Marie Claire* and no other monthly women's magazine. However, this is dodgy territory and if you're going to stretch the boundaries of exclusivity, you need to make sure everyone concerned is very clear about the deal.

Publicist James Herring is well versed in helping ordinary people who suddenly find themselves in the media spotlight. He handled all the publicity for the first series of Channel 4's Big Brother. *He warns potential kiss and tellers:*

'Be extremely cautious! I think you should always think long and hard before hanging your dirty washing in public for money.

'By selling your story for money, you are inviting people into your personal life and it's hard to reclaim it.

'Bear in mind the long-term consequences; you might have £15,000 in your bank account, but you're fair game for any media which might want to find out the other side of the story.

'If you hire a publicist to help you make money from your story, they'll be working on a commission. They'll push their fee up by asking you to talk more about a certain area – particularly if your story is a kiss and tell. They might persuade you to pose for some provocative photographs which could embarrass you further down the line.

'There's a big difference between a PR agent who's there to say how using the media will benefit you over a period of time, and somebody who's there to make a quick buck.'

Real
LIFE

If publications are really badgering you for an exclusive – or you have lots to say or show – you might be able to offer different exclusives to each. You might give one an exclusive picture, while the other gets an exclusive interview. But be careful with this – you're playing with fire.

Not every story has to be an exclusive but don't send a story to one newspaper and then expect another to run the same story a week or a month later. If they know it's appeared elsewhere previously, they'll tell you where to go. If they don't know and they run the story themselves, and *then* they find out, they'll never speak to you again.

IT'S NOT NEWS – BUT IS IT STILL WORTH READING?

Your story might, of course, not be 'hard' enough to make the news pages – it simply might not be news. But that doesn't mean you're dead in the water. You might still be able to get your story in print. It might be suitable to be one of the following, and you should look through your chosen publication – there might be other categories.

FEATURE General longer article. In newspapers, features are usually carried after the news pages.

REGULAR Look through your target publication and see if your story might fit into one of their regular features; they might run a 'How to …' or 'Ask the expert' section.

PROFILE Special interview with interesting person – you! Trade papers are particularly fond of profiles. Sometimes they might also do company profiles, about a firm rather than an individual.

OP-ED PIECES/COLUMNS Mid-length articles that are very personal and opinionated.

LETTERS TO THE EDITOR

HOW TO HANDLE THAT PHONE CALL.

Phew, we're back on the speaking bit now. You've thought about your story, written your press release and sent it to just the right person. They were delighted to hear from you and they want to interview you.

OR, you've decided that a press release isn't appropriate and it's better to call them.

OR, they've heard about *you* and want to chat.

FINDING YOUR CENTRAL MESSAGE

Before you open your mouth to speak to anyone, make sure you know what you want to say.

Think about your story and imagine you only have 20 seconds to make your point. What would you say?

>> p13

What am I trying to achieve?

If you're struggling, why not have a look at the section in chapter 1 which deals with finding your Objective and End Result.

DO sit down and write a list of your key points. Then be ruthless. Keep crossing off the points until you find your Objective and End Result.

DO keep them at the forefront of your mind throughout all your dealings with the media.

DO remind yourself of your Objective and End Result if you falter in your interview, and you'll be back on track.

IF YOU'RE CALLING THEM OUT OF THE BLUE

The first and most important thing is to make sure you've got the timing right – if you haven't read the section 'Get the timing right' on page 180, have a scan through it first. When phoning, timing is even more important. The time of your call can make all the difference between a friendly chat and a curt exchange.

Daily newspapers often have much shorter deadlines – although even they plan features and supplements way ahead of time. But shorter deadlines mean more intense deadlines. Ring reception and ask what is a good time to call a journalist.

Most national newspapers have their main news meeting at around 11 am. If you have a piece of news for the following day's paper, call the journalist before 11 am, so they can put your story on the main news list.

After that, the best time to call is between about 12 noon and 2.30 pm. Later, news journalists tend to come under pressure from deadlines and won't be so free to talk. Also, the later you leave it, the harder it is to squeeze stories in to the following day's paper.

Features writers are generally more flexible – call any time from around 10 am.

WHATEVER YOU DO, DON'T PHONE WITH NON-URGENT NEWS AROUND 11 am.

DON'T try to engage them in a friendly chat unless they start it.

DON'T fix meetings if you could have told them over the phone or in an email.

DO suggest lunch or a drink and then leave it up to them if you're keen to set up a relationship.

DO remember that most journalists are being pulled in 1,001 directions.

Get prepared – even if you've written a press release, have that in front of you. If you've decided not to write one, jot down what you want to say – nerves can often make you stammer, stutter and wander off the subject.

WHAT IF THEY CALL YOU?

James Herring suggests: *'If you're planning to phone a journalist, or you are expecting a call from the press, sit down first and write down exactly what you want to get across.*

'But if a journalist calls you, never feel you have to give an immediate response. It's fine to say you'll call back. You can ask them to give you all their questions over the phone, and say you'll call back with your response. The fact that you did will never appear in print and is a perfectly reasonable practice.'

In 99.99 per cent of cases, if a journalist calls *you*, it will be about something perfectly innocent. However, they might well be up against a deadline and putting pressure on you to answer their questions immediately. If you can, all well and good, but if you feel your personal or business reputation is at stake, you have a right to ask for a few minutes to consider your answer.

Ask the journalist to give you all the questions they're planning to ask, note them down, then ask them what the deadline is. Collect your thoughts – maybe make a few notes – and call back as soon as you can.

Keep your answers clear and to the point – if they don't ask you about a point you consider important, don't forget to bring it up yourself, and explain why it's so vital. If you are being interviewed for a news story, a journalist will normally take about 10 or 15 minutes to chat to you over the phone.

If a longer feature is planned, the journalist may want to meet you face to face. If they do conduct the interview over the phone, you might be talking for around 45 minutes, although it really depends on the publication and the subject-matter.

HELP!

I've got something to hide and I don't want to talk to any journalists.

If you possibly can, it's always better to give journalists something, rather than nothing. Saying 'no comment' comes across badly. The public view the words suspiciously and wonder what you've got to hide.

If the reporter really has hit a raw nerve, or they are questioning you about something that really must remain secret, the best thing to do is to prepare a statement. You already know that you don't have to answer questions immediately. Take the journalist's number, find out their deadline and prepare a statement. Keep it brief and unambiguous.

If the subject is legally sensitive, you might want to consult a lawyer before speaking.

'I regret that, for legal reasons, I am unable to comment on the rumours ...'

'I'm sorry, but it's company policy not to comment on speculation about financial matters.'

These are both reasonable responses. Look in any newspaper and you'll see real-life examples.

If you can't talk about an issue yet, but will be able to later, offer to let the journalist know when you can discuss it.

DON'T agree to call back and then never do so.

DON'T simply make yourself unavailable.

DO ask someone else to call back and read your statement to the journalist. Even if you give a statement, a journalist will still try to wheedle more out of you. If you don't think you'll be able to remain strong in the face of such questioning, by all means ask someone else to act as your spokesperson.

And, whatever else you do, DON'T LIE!

Never, ever, ever lie to the media.

James Herring says: *'Never lie to the media. You cannot lie to the media without it bouncing back to get you sooner or later. If you get found out – and you will – you'll lose everyone's respect, including the respect of any media who might have considered you a trustworthy source in the future. You'll have blown your opportunity.'*

SIMPLE DOS & DONT'S

DO tell the truth.

DO make sure the journalist or interviewer knows how to spell and pronounce your name.

DO make sure the journalist or interviewer knows your job title and company, or your position within the campaign – whatever background information is appropriate.

DO prepare for any interview by thinking about what questions are likely to be asked.

DO mug up on facts and figures – have them written down if you think you might forget.

DO try to chat to the interviewer or journalist beforehand, to make sure they're au fait with the subject.

DON'T try to tell them anything off the record – this is very dangerous and different people sometimes have different interpretations of what 'off the record' means.

DON'T ask to see the copy before it is published or broadcast. Most journalists will be highly offended by this. If they want you to see it – or any part of it – to check matters of fact, they'll ask you.

DON'T let your emotions get the better of you – especially anger and especially if it's directed at the journalist. If your story is sad and you become upset, that's different, but take a deep breath and try to pull yourself together – you're there because you have something to say – don't waste your opportunity. Cry all you like after the interview.

DON'T criticise those who disagree with you. Name-calling just comes across as childish and will take the focus away from the issues.

DO retain good manners and good humour throughout, however rattled you might be.

MAKING THE MOST OF YOUR MEDIA TIME

● Think before you speak – as with any form of public speaking, your adrenalin will be rushing about. A pause may seem like an age to you, but is likely to come across as thoughtfulness to the audience or the reporter.

- Keep it short – if you can make it catchy, so much the better. All journalists love a sound bite.

- If you have something technical, medical or otherwise complicated to explain, think about how you can do this in simple language, but without being patronising.

- Avoid jargon, obscure references or acronyms.

- Try not to get dragged into meaningless hypothetical discussions – 'what if's – just discuss the here and now.

- Talk about your area of expertise and then shut up. Don't be dragged into subjects you don't know a lot about.

- If the journalist gets something wrong when they're asking you a question, correct the mistake then answer the question.

- Answer the question you want to answer. If you're asked a mischievous question, rephrase it into something you're happy with. Don't fumble about because someone asks you the equivalent of 'When did you stop beating your wife?'.

- If they keep on at you, repeating the question, keep on repeating your answer. You may change the words, but make it clear that you're simply reinforcing your point.

- Make sure you say important names – like the name of your company or organisation.

- If you're acting as a spokesperson for your company, organisation or campaign, reporters and the public won't distinguish between your personal opinion and the opinion of the organisation you represent. Don't get drawn into giving your personal opinions.

JARGONBUSTER!

Sound bite: a short extract of recorded (now also reported) speech which is particularly catchy and quotable. It tends to sum up a situation or feeling in just a few words.

EXAMPLES OF SOUND BITES

'Ask not what your country can do for you, rather what you can do for your country'

'She was the People's Princess'

'There were three people in that marriage'

'I have a dream'

DON'T work up to your point – work backwards. Say the most important thing first and then fill in the background if you get the chance.

DON'T give one-word answers – it'll look as if you have something to hide, or at the very least like you're being awkward.

DON'T guess or bluff. If you don't know, say so – but say you'll try to find out.

DON'T refuse to answer unless you can help it. If you can't help it, explain why you can't answer the question: there's a legal reason; there are market sensitivities; it's too early to say, etc.

SPECIAL ADVICE FOR TELEVISION AND RADIO

Although the preceding advice has concentrated on newspapers and the rest of the printed press, pretty much all of it applies equally to television and radio. If you're being interviewed for a news piece, you'll probably only be on camera for five or ten minutes. The crew may well prefer to come to you for the filming – which at least gives you a home advantage. Although the interview will be over quickly, it can take some time to set up lights and angles, etc. Make sure you allow plenty of time for the interview. Radio interviews are usually done over the phone, and often take only five or ten minutes.

If you are asked to go to the television or radio studios, the researcher (or whoever you speak to) should be able to give you an idea of how long you'll be there. But don't schedule a vital meeting immediately afterwards – these things invariably over-run.

As well as finding out how long it should take, find out everything you can about the programme concerned.

Then ask yourself:

● Do I understand exactly what's expected of me?

● Can I speak knowledgeably on this subject?

Rehearse your answers, rope in friends, family or colleagues as sounding boards, and tape yourself.

● If you're appearing on the radio, a simple tape recorder will do.

● If you're going on television, try to borrow or hire a video camera.

TIP
You're the expert on your topic. Be confident. Keep your tone of voice conversational.

CHECKLIST

Ask yourself the following questions:

Firstly, and rather obviously, which programme is
inviting me to speak? If you're not familiar with the
programme, ask for tapes. ❏

Is it live or pre-recorded? ❏

How long will the interview take? ❏

Where will the recording take place? If you're unfamiliar
with the location, ask if they'll send a car for you –
or plan your route carefully and allow plenty of time. ❏

What time do I need to be there? ❏

When will the programme be broadcast, and on
which channel or station? ❏

Who will be interviewing me? ❏

Will I meet the interviewer beforehand? ❏

Are there other people being interviewed? Who are they?
If you don't know the other panellists, or
interviewees, ask for a biog, or more information. ❏

Am I being pitted against the other interviewee
as presenting two opposing arguments? ❏

>> p97

Your voice

>> p104

What should I do with my body?

● Play the tape back and look at it with a critical eye. If you have a problem with your voice, see the section on 'Your voice' in chapter 6.

● If you have odd physical mannerisms, look up the relevant sections in chapter 6.

DON'T read from a prepared statement. Assume you're being taped from the moment you get there until the moment you leave.

DON'T ramble on but give them enough material to use.

DO practise answering questions in 20 seconds or less. They'll probably use 20-second chunks anyway, so practise squeezing your message into these chunks.

DO practice what you want to say.

DO correct any mistakes politely and try not to be fazed by interruptions. Ask to be allowed to finish and give a proper answer to the question.

DON'T argue with the reporter. Correct mistakes but keep a sense of perspective. Often, the reporter will have been instructed to try to wind you up. Don't fall for it!

DON'T waffle. When you've answered a question, shut up. It's hugely tempting to blather on to avoid silence, but don't!

DON'T answer a question with a question. If you're asked, 'What do you think about educating disabled children alongside the able-bodied?', don't say, 'What do you mean by disabled?' Either you'll sound aggressive or evasive.

DO take a deep breath and start your answer again if you're not being interviewed live and you make a mistake. It will seem weird but they will be able to edit out the first attempt. Don't ruin this by apologising at length. (I bet the interviewer fluffs at least one question and he's supposed to be the professional!)

DON'T worry if they ask you to run through your answer two, three or even more times. It happens all the time and they won't lose patience. Honestly! It might not even be your fault – there might be a problem with the equipment. Be grateful that you'll have several opportunities to practise making your point.

DO simply stop and say 'I'm sorry, I haven't answered that very well – let me try again' if you make a mistake when you're being interviewed live. They've invited you there to put across your point of view, so they'll be pleased if you do so clearly and concisely.

I worked in television for several years and I've been to many recordings and shoots. Even the most professional, experienced and admired presenters make mistakes – all the time. And even if you're an avid fan of *It'll Be Alright On The Night,* you'd still be shocked if you could see how many takes are needed to get something right. After a while, presenters stop worrying and just concentrate on getting it right. Take a leaf out of their book and make mistakes like a pro!

SPECIAL TV TIPS

Get there early but expect to start late and finish late. TV is *always* late. But they'll scream blue murder if *you're* late. Check the following for help on what to wear.

Dress smartly from head to toe, just in case they film a long shot of you. But remember that the camera will probably only focus on your head and shoulders – don't wear anything fussy, revealing (unless you're doing it on purpose) or bulky. Stick to simple lines. Wear something that's comfortable.

Avoid very short skirts – you might be seated for the interview. At best, it could be unflattering (squashed-up cellulite never looks good). At worst you could 'do a Sharon Stone', if you know what I mean. Also avoid bright colours – they might clash with the set and jump out at the viewer – and never wear busy patterns, or contrasty stripes and small checks – the camera won't be able to cope and you'll look like a bizarre kind of kaleidoscope. Don't wear high contrasts like black and white, for the same reason.

Plain colours in flattering, soft shades are best. Black can make you look like you're in mourning – viewers switching on halfway through might think a member of the royal family has died, or something. Avoid too much jewellery – noises that in real life sound like tinkles and clinks will be amplified into clunking great crashes that will drown out your words of wisdom.

Remember Tony Blair at the 2000 Labour Party conference: TV lights are hot stuff and they make you sweat. Wear deodorant, choose a lightweight suit and if you have a real tendency to perspire, wear a plain white T-shirt under your shirt. It will soak up a lot of yukky sweat.

Empty your pockets – odd bulges will only look worse on television – and if you're wearing a tie, straighten it. If you're wearing trousers, make sure your socks are long enough so you're not showing a flash of leg. Make sure your shirt is tucked in. Turn off your mobile or pager – or leave it in another room.

WHAT ABOUT HAIR AND MAKEUP?

Make sure your hair is clean, and style it so it's off your face. Overlong fringes or weird wispy bits will throw funny shadows and the viewers will think you're ready for Hallowe'en.

Just wear your normal makeup – if you need more, they'll organise that. If you're a man, they'll powder you if you're looking shiny, so don't worry.

HELP! MY BODY HAS TURNED AGAINST ME!

VOICE See the section on 'Your voice' in chapter 6.

>> p97

Your voice

The sound man will ask you to speak so that he can get his 'levels'.

Now is the time to use your normal voice at its normal level. And sit in the position you're going to sit in during the interview.

It doesn't really matter what you say to set your level – no one cares. Most people say their name and where they're from. Some say a few lines of a nursery rhyme or poem.

JARGONBUSTER!

Levels: sound equipment has gauges that show the amount of sound being picked up. The sound man can set each microphone to the right level, so that you'll be heard properly, without deafening anyone.

During the interview, try to sit more or less still, without looking as if you're practising for musical statues. The levels have been set, so there's no need to lean into the mike. If your voice is wavering about because of nerves, try some of the relaxation and breathing exercises in this book.

HANDS If you're sitting at a desk, put your hands on top of it. If you don't have a desk but you're sitting down, fold your hands in your lap – hiding your hands will at best make you look shifty; at worst like you're fiddling with yourself.

If you're standing up, don't cross your arms. Hands in pockets can look casual – maybe too casual, depending on the circumstances. If you feel really uncomfortable, try holding a book, or file, or something relevant. If you still feel uncomfortable, ask if you can do the interview sitting down.

DON'T be afraid to gesticulate. But,

DON'T wave your fist, point or make any rude signs. It comes across terribly badly on television.

LEGS Sit up straight. Don't swivel about. If you cross your legs, it will make your thighs look fat. And if you uncross them on camera, you'll look like that Kenny Everett character who waved 'her' legs around like a windmill. Or like Sharon Stone in *Fatal Attraction*. This might be a good idea if you're launching a career as a topless model but isn't so wise for the rest of us.

DO either cross your legs at the ankles or keep your feet together, sliding one slightly ahead of the other. A good trick is to swivel your knees to one side – it's the most flattering way to sit.

DO lean forward very slightly in your chair. Slouching back will make you look uninterested or afraid.

DO try sitting in front of a mirror in your chosen outfit – find the best way to sit and make sure your slip isn't going to show.

DON'T leap to your feet as soon as you've finished speaking. We've all seen that done and it's excruciating. Just sit still, exactly where you are and look poised.

DON'T face squarely on to the camera if you do have to stand. If you swivel your body round slightly, you will look slimmer – and don't forget, the camera adds about 10 pounds, so most of us need all the help we can get!

Here's how to do it:

- Stand with your right foot in front of the other.
- Imagine your feet are the hands of a clock – but six inches or so apart.
- Point your right foot to 12 o'clock.
- Point your left foot to 10 o'clock.
- Put slightly more weight on your right foot (you can switch this around to the other side, if you feel more comfortable).

This stance is very solid, so you'll look slim *and* you won't fall over. Bonus!

TORSO Don't sway or rock, and keep your shoulders back.

HEAD Hold it high and don't wave it about. Nod if you agree, by all means.

EYES Look at the journalist – pay attention at all times, because if the camera picks up your wandering gaze, it will make you look shifty. Unless you're looking up at the sky, which will make you look like you're pleading with God. Or you're looking at the ground, which will make you look like you're either asleep or praying. And *never* try to look into the camera. It will make you look like a newsreader. Or Uri Geller.

DON'T gaze around the studio (however fascinating it might be and however many people are running around).

DON'T avoid eye contact with the journalist.

DO wear your glasses if you need to. The lighting man will fix it so there's not too much glare from the lenses. But you won't be able to wear photochromic lenses because they'll just go dark as soon as the lights go on and you'll look like an ageing Hollywood star or a boxer the morning after the fight.

ENTIRE BODY If you feel like you've lost control of your entire body, it's probably stress. As opposed to St Vitus's Dance or some kind of fit. Be aware of how you behave during stress – you might need to ask someone else. If you're aware that you normally tap your foot, fiddle with your hair or grimace, you'll be less likely to do it.

DEALING WITH DIFFICULT QUESTIONS

As I've already said, the overwhelming majority of journalists are honest and accurate.

But there are a few bad apples – if your subject has anything to do with politics, you might find yourself on the opposite side to the journalist, for example. Although they are supposed to be unbiased, some can't and others simply won't be. There are also times when even good journalists might feel the need to give you a hard time. Let's go through some of the tricky bits.

LOADED QUESTIONS

The journalist builds his case by making a number of statements and then comes in with the killer: the loaded question.

'The local education authorities have suffered a major cutback in funding this year. Most schools don't have enough books or computer equipment. Why should we spend so much money adapting one village school for one child?'

WHAT SHOULD I SAY? Start by either rejecting or accepting the statements and then link to your Objective.

'In fact, local authorities have been given additional grants for computer equipment, which frees cash for other areas of spending this year. However, we accept that they are not prepared to spend the money on these adaptations. But we think there's an important issue at the heart of this – and that's the right of physically disabled children to be part of mainstream education. And that's why we've launched the fund-raising campaign – so that Kerry, and other children like her, can go to the school of their choice.'

HOBSON'S CHOICE

The reporter asks you to choose between two extremes, neither of which is desirable.

'Would you prefer the licence fee to be spent on obscure arts programmes that fall into the public service remit or should the BBC devote the cash to popular shows that win big audiences?'

WHAT SHOULD I SAY? Don't feel you have to plump for one or the other. Say you reject both arguments and return to your Objective.

'Neither of those options is acceptable on its own. As part of the BBC's public service remit, it has to serve all kinds of audiences and we feel we distribute the licence fee effectively. Just because a programme has a smaller audience, it doesn't mean we shouldn't serve that audience. We just need to be as sensible as we've always been.'

HYPOTHETICALS

The reporter creates a hypothetical situation and follows up with a question.

'Imagine a big multinational company has offered to donate £10,000 to your environment group, but you know they are one of the biggest polluters in the area?'

WHAT SHOULD I SAY? Don't get pulled into the hypothetical – you could end up tying yourself in knots. Revert to your Objective if possible.

'Nothing like that has ever happened. You seem to be asking about where we get our funds from. Our members pay an annual subscription and help us by staging fund-raising events. These moneys and any other donations are clearly shown in our accounts, which can be viewed by anyone at our website – Environment.com.'

THE DOG WITH A BONE

The reporter won't give it up and keeps coming back to you with the same question.

'But what if they really offered you a lot of money? Wouldn't it be immoral to refuse?'

WHAT SHOULD I SAY? Don't fall into the trap of giving them what they want, either to make them happy or to shut them up. Rephrase your answer if you want, but remember your Objective.

'I can't really comment on situations that don't exist. We are entirely open about our funding and always strive to work towards our aim of protecting the environment. That's our main concern – and at the moment we're particularly concerned about the amount of pollution in the sea and the filth washing up on British beaches.'

COMMENT ON A COMMENT ON A COMMENT

Stories can sometimes spin out of control because no one has bothered to find out the true facts, which are now buried under a mountain of hype, misquotes and misinformation.

'What do you think about Fred Benson's accusation that you are out of touch and inefficient?'

WHAT SHOULD I SAY? If you didn't directly hear someone make a particular comment, don't be drawn into commenting on it yourself. The comments may have been taken out of context. Try to go back to your Objective.

'Fred has certainly never said anything like that to me! I've worked with Fred for years and if he has any criticisms I'm sure he wouldn't hold back in coming and saying them straight to me!' Then link back to your Objective.

UNITED WE STAND!

A journalist might try to cause trouble by exposing (or creating) a split within your organisation.

'Don't you think £2 million is a hell of a lot to have spent on the brand-new office building?'

WHAT SHOULD I SAY? If you're not the expert on a particular area, say so. If asked about something that falls into a colleague's remit, refer the journalist back to the right person.

'I only control my own budget – you'd have to speak to Malcolm Williams about the new office! I do know that Malcolm has substantially increased my own budget this year and I'm delighted that it's meant I can invest in 200 extra hours of programming, including a fantastic adaptation of *Wuthering Heights*, which starts next Sunday at 8 pm.'

THAT'S JUST PLAIN WRONG!

The reporter asks you a question based on totally incorrect information, or information you perceive as wrong.

'When are schools going to get the funding they deserve?'

WHAT SHOULD I SAY? Correct them straight away, or the audience might accept the information or inference. Go back to your Objective.

'I'm convinced that schools already receive a good level of funding. The budget went up 15 per cent above inflation this year and we've been able to equip 15 more schools with brand-new computer equipment.'

THE TWISTER

The reporter twists your words to turn them back on you.

'You mean our children have been struggling with poor equipment until now?'

WHAT SHOULD I SAY? Restate your comment, or expand on it, so there's no misunderstanding.

'Let me make myself clear: school equipment in our area is already well above the national average. But the extra money has meant we've achieved our target of having five pupils to each computer. The national average is eight pupils per computer.'

DON'T PUT WORDS IN MY MOUTH!

Don't repeat negative words. Journalists sometimes ask aggressive and negative questions.

'Many people have complained that the standard of teaching today is appalling. What do you say to them?'

WHAT SHOULD I SAY? Well, what you *shouldn't* say is, '*I don't think the standard of teaching is appalling.*' They could edit out the question and it will sound as if you brought it up. Always turn it round and emphasise the positive.

'You'll see from the last set of exam results that pupils are getting higher grades than ever before.'

ONE THING AFTER ANOTHER

The reporter asks you a whole lot of questions, all at once.

WHAT SHOULD I SAY? Just answer the one you want to answer – the one that will link most easily to your Objective.

INTERRUPTING

The journalist fires another question while you're only halfway through answering the previous one.

WHAT SHOULD I SAY? Don't forget the rule that you should always be polite. Just ask that you be allowed to finish answering the last question first.

DEAD AIR

You finish your answer but the reporter says nothing and there's a big, fat embarrassing silence.

WHAT SHOULD I SAY? Nothing at all. They're controlling the interview so it's their problem. If you really feel uncomfortable, why not say: 'Does that answer your question?'

THE KNOCK

The reporter comes to your house or your office and either knocks on your door or ambushes you just outside.

WHAT SHOULD I SAY? We've all seen this on the television – on *Watchdog* and *Roger Cook*, etc. What do you think of the people who run away? You think they're scoundrels with something to hide, right? And what about the people who answer pleasantly, or appear

> **TIP**
> No matter how hot your story, always remember, the press is doing you a favour, not the other way round. Don't call them saying: 'I'd like to place a story with you' or 'I'd like some editorial'.

later in the studio? You might think they've done something wrong, but you don't think they're crooks. They'll probably try to put it right.

If you get ambushed, resist the temptation to run away. It doesn't matter how busy or surprised you are, turn and face the journalist.

Use the tips for when a journalist phones you out of the blue – ask them what they want, what questions they need to ask and when they need to hear from you. Tell them when you'll be able to get back to them – AND DO IT.

If you really can't discuss the matter, call the journalist and tell them you are going to issue a statement (see above for tips on making a statement). You can either read this on camera or to the mike, or you can simply send it to the journalist. For reporters from newspapers or magazines it's obviously fine to send a written statement. For broadcast media, it's better to appear on camera, or, for radio, read the statement to the reporter. Be firm about supplementary questions and say, 'I'm sorry, I've given you my statement. I really can't say any more about it at this stage, for the reasons I've already mentioned. I'll be happy to talk to you further when this becomes public.'

If you can grant an interview and you're confident about handling it then and there, why not invite the journalist in? You will look much more professional if you are interviewed at your desk, on home territory, than if you give an interview in the car park, with your hair being blown about by the wind and with your hands full of papers, briefcase and mobile phone. By inviting the reporter in, you are also giving a subliminal message that you have nothing to hide.

They have tried to surprise you, but you can take control of the situation.

It's not uncommon for reporters to ambush a news source outside their office or home. Respond as if the reporter had called you on the phone. You might ask what the story is about and when they need the information. Tell the reporter when you or someone else will be able to get back to them. You are not obligated to consent to the ambush interview if you are unprepared or the time is inconvenient.

HMM, THAT'S A TOUGHIE!
The journalist asks you a very difficult question – it's not that you don't know the answer, it's finding the right way to say it.

WHAT SHOULD I SAY? Simply pause for thought. As we have discovered before, pauses seem worse to you than to anyone listening. If you're being interviewed for a newspaper, the reporter can't *write* a pause. And they're unlikely even to mention that you paused.

And if you are doing a recorded broadcast interview, pauses are usually edited out.

Even if it is live, you'll simply look thoughtful. Which you are. The chances are, the audience will recognise that it's a difficult subject and they'll respect you for giving it due thought.

EMERGENCIES, ACCIDENTS & INCIDENTS

It may be that your company is somehow involved in an accident – a gas explosion in the office, for example. I know these are horrible thoughts but you might be involved in an accident – or you might witness a crime or a crash.

You might be a member of the services, called to a major incident and it suddenly falls to you to speak to the waiting press.

Whatever the emergency, it's a difficult situation. Emotions may be running high – if people are injured, survivors and relatives will be angry and looking for someone to blame. The media will be on even tighter deadlines than usual and the niceties might go straight out of the window.

Keep a cool head, remember a few golden rules and you'll get through.

SHOULDN'T I BE DOING SOMETHING MORE USEFUL?
In an emergency, you might feel that you'd be better off elsewhere – and you might also think the media would be better off elsewhere – anywhere except here, making matters worse! You might rather be in the thick of things, carrying on helping people. You might rather be with your colleagues, finding out what the hell went wrong. You might rather be at the hospital, finding out if your own friends or family are all right.

But if you're there in an official capacity (not just as a witness), you really are doing something useful if you're making the necessary statement to the press.

Remember that relatives might be worried and they're going to get their information from the media. If they don't hear what's going on, they too might come to the scene and hamper the rescue or clean-up.

Give the media clear, concise, regular messages to keep them off your back and give everyone the information to which they have a right.

If the emergency services are involved, special systems will swing into action and phone lines will be manned by spokespeople. But journalists will always prefer to speak to someone at the scene than to a trained spokesperson in a cosy warm office.

They will grab witnesses, bystanders, survivors – anyone. And sometimes rumour and conjecture can dramatically exaggerate the scale of the problem. Keep things under control by giving calm, factual briefings whenever you have new information.

PEOPLE ARE NUMBER ONE

Whatever has happened, remember that people should be your number one concern. Mention victims or survivors first and decline to comment about other matters, such as money.

If someone has been injured, her mother won't thank you for talking about how much it's going to cost you to sort out the damage.

BE REALISTIC

Just as you shouldn't allow an accident to be hyped out of control by rumours and speculation, don't try to play down a tragedy.

DON'T SPECULATE

As soon as there's an accident of any kind, reporters will want to know if anyone was hurt and how badly. The second thing they'll want to know is how it happened.

DON'T get drawn into speculation. Simply say that you are investigating as a matter of urgency and you will let them know as soon as there are any conclusions.

The public enquiries for the rail disasters of the last few years have made their reports months and even years after the tragedies. In the aftermath of accidents – such as the Concorde crash in Paris – the newspapers are full of possible causes. But if *you* jump the gun and start speculating, you may look foolish or cause more panic.

DON'T BLAME INDIVIDUALS OR GROUPS

This is an extension of the previous point. Don't attempt to lay blame with anyone personally. Don't discuss previous incidents or problems. If these are relevant, they will emerge in the fullness of time. If they're not, you risk a serious libel action.

If someone in your company or organisation has been arrested, do not discuss their previous behaviour record. Such information could prejudice a fair trial and you'll find yourself in the dock, too.

DO say: 'I have a story you might be interested in' or 'I'm going to send you my biog. I just wanted to let you know that if you're doing any stories about x, I might be able to help, or comment.'

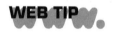

My favourite place for links to sites packed with media tips is www.newsbureau.com.

SUMMARY

If you don't get much coverage, don't be disheartened. Think about why your story or interview wasn't used, or was cut to almost nothing.

If you really, hand on heart, think you've done everything right, remember there might have been another reason.

It might have been a busy news day; the next time might be a slow day. The subject-matter might have been unfashionable; it might come back into the spotlight (or you could make it more current). The news editor who was on duty that day might not have liked it, but their colleague might love it and will run your next story. You might have happened upon one of the editor's pet hates. The journalist might have filed a badly written story because they had a headache – they'll get better. The sub-editor might have been having a bad day.

But don't be put off.

James Herring says: *'Ultimately, journalists are in the business of finding news and entertaining their readership. You shouldn't be scared of approaching them with your story.*

'This is especially true if you want to talk to them about your business, or a charity venture. Most journalists will be very glad to hear from you.

'Usually someone, somewhere will want to know your story – even if it's a straightforward "local boy done good" piece for your local paper.

'And once you've got it in print, it's much easier to get in print again.

'Don't be scared of the media – use it. It's there for you.'

11
PROBLEMS AND
TROUBLESHOOTING

* LIBEL & SLANDER

* HECKLING

* NERVES

* PROBLEMS WITH THE VENUE

* WHEN MACHINERY LETS YOU DOWN

This is the chapter to read if you've got problems. Well, with public speaking anyway. It's a general rule of life that if something can go wrong, it will. Don't be disheartened. There is seldom a problem that can't be sorted out with a little thought and enough determination.

Many of the problems you might encounter have been covered in previous chapters, but it does no harm to recap and stress that you can overcome them!

LIBEL & SLANDER

The law on libel and slander – collectively known as 'defamation' – is so complicated that this book can only give you a rough guide to the main pitfalls. If you're anxious to say something and you're concerned it could be defamatory, make an appointment to see your nearest friendly libel lawyer.

WHAT DOES 'DEFAMATION' MEAN?

The lawyer-speak definition of defamation is that the law recognises that every woman/man has the right to have the estimation in which he stands in the opinion of others unaffected by false and defamatory statements and imputations.

Stripped down to the bare minimum, it covers anything said or written about a person that makes you think less of him/her.

A defamatory statement is one which does one of the following to the person it's about:

1 exposes them to hatred, ridicule or contempt

2 causes them to be shunned or avoided

3 lowers them in the estimation of right-thinking members of society generally

4 disparages them in their business, trade, office or profession

If it's written down (or permanent, such as a picture), it's libel. If it's spoken it's slander. The only exceptions are that defamatory statements made on television, radio or in a play count as libel.

The trouble with the definition of libel is that no one has been able to think up a form of words that explains it all properly, covering all eventualities. One of the main problems relates to that phrase in point 3: 'right-thinking members of society generally'. When a lawyer is deciding whether something is defamatory, they try to think what this imaginary person might possibly think. And with changing times comes a changing 'right-thinking' person. What was defamatory 20 years ago might not be so now. So you can see how these things are open to different interpretations.

As I said before, this is a hugely complicated legal issue – far too complicated to go into here. Just beware that even repeating something that's already been said on television or written in a newspaper could find you in extremely hot water.

If you want to know more about slander, and defamation laws in general, try *McNae's Essential Law for Journalists*, published by Butterworths, for a concise no-nonsense explanation.

HECKLING

See chapter 7, page 114, 'Dealing with difficult people'.

NERVES

See chapter 6, page 89, Nerves.

PROBLEMS WITH THE VENUE

See chapter 5, page 78, 'Coping with the venue'.

WHEN MACHINERY LETS YOU DOWN

See chapter 4, page 48, 'Words are not enough'.

12
CONCLUSION

Well, good luck with it. I hope this book has helped boost your speaking confidence – and given you a few new ideas and tips to help.

If you only bought it in the hope of making your point more clearly in meetings, I hope your horizons are now somewhat wider.

Remember – there's nothing to it!

At the very beginning of the book, I gave you a tip and told you to remember it, even if you forgot everything else:

Who? What? Why? When? Where? How?

Well, I'm actually going to ask you to remember one more tip, as well. It's my best public speaking tip, boiled right down to its simplest form. It's just:

STAND UP, SPEAK UP and SHUT UP.